Competition and Monopoly in Medical Care

Competition and Monopoly in Medical Care

H. E. Frech III

The AEI Press

Publisher for the American Enterprise Institute
WASHINGTON, D.C.

1996

Available in the United States from the AEI Press, c/o Publisher Resources, Inc., 1224 Heil Quaker Blvd., P.O. Box 7001, La Vergne, TN 37086-7001. Distributed outside the United States by arrangement with Eurospan, 3 Henrietta Street, London WC2E 8LU England.

Library of Congress Cataloging-in-Publication Data

Frech, H. E.
    Competition and monopoly in medical care / H. E. Frech III.
        p.   cm.
    Includes bibliographical references and index.
    ISBN 0-8447-3884-0 (cloth).—ISBN 0-8447-3885-9 (paper)
    1. Medical economics.   2. Competition.   I. Title.
RA410.5.F74   1996
362.1—dc20   96-11636
                                                          CIP

1   3   5   7   9   10   8   6   4   2

Printed in the United States of America

This book is dedicated to Liz, Michael, Justin, and Clayton.

Contents

Preface

I wrote this book for several audiences. I hope that the small core of specialists in medical care competition will find the book a valuable summary and reference and will find my interpretations and suggestions generally convincing and sometimes provocative.

But there are two additional audiences for this book. One is economists who are not specialists in health care. Nonspecialist economists should find the book a useful introduction to health care competition and health economics.

The second audience is noneconomists with an interest in health care policy and some background in basic economics. (Knowledge of supply-and-demand analysis and competitive and monopoly equilibriums is helpful.) Health care specialists should find the book a helpful explanation of how economists analyze competition.

Because my intended audience includes nonspecialists in health care, I have made the exposition as accessible as possible to those with little background in economics, mathematics, or statistics. Only a few equations can be found, mostly in appendixes or footnotes for interested readers. Readers may cheerfully ignore them. This approach is not a serious disadvantage for the specialist. Making sense of the sprawling literature and disparate empirical results requires theoretical and empirical judgment. Formal model building and advanced econometric testing are important research approaches but are not so useful in a synthesis such as this.

The main focus of the book is positive economics, not normative economics. That is, the book deals with how the health economy works, not so much with how it should work or what policies would be best. Whether more competition is good or bad is only covered occasionally and incidentally. The concluding chapter addresses this topic in more detail. This approach reflects the literature. Not much analytical or empirical literature touches directly the overarching policy issue, even though much research is motivated by policy concerns. At the same time, that increasing competition is, on balance, good will be clear to readers.

For a general textbook on health economics, see Charles E. Phelps

(1992, *Health Economics*); Sherman Folland, Allen C. Goodman, and Miron Stano (1993, *The Economics of Health and Health Care*); or Paul J. Feldstein (1979, *Health Care Economics*). The focus is on health care competition and monopoly. Many policy and research topics not closely related to this focus are excluded.

Many people helped with this project. My colleague Llad Phillips urged me to write the book based on themes from my earlier writings. Helpful research assistance was provided by Paul Murphy, Clayton Frech, and Ken Danger. Lee Mobley, Colin Day, Jongkee Hong, Theodore Keeler, Will Manning, Mark Perlman, Robert Helms, and Richard Scheffler provided excellent criticism of earlier drafts.

Competition and Monopoly in Medical Care

1
Introduction

Competition in health care has grown rapidly in recent years, both in fact and in theory. Actual competition has grown with reforms in private health insurance and a weakening of professional power. Monopolistic elements in health care, though still important, have receded. As a topic for study and research, competition has grown even faster. The study of competition is itself a growth area. The literature is large, diverse, but poorly connected. A critical survey and synthesis are missing.

This book is designed to fill that need, to explain what we know, mostly from the research literature, about how competition and monopoly function in the health care sector. The role of competition in this market is controversial and debatable. This book is meant to contribute to that debate indirectly by raising the level of scientific understanding underlying the policy discussions. The book is not meant to be polemical. Though my own preference for competition in health care surfaces, this is primarily a work of positive economics, not normative economics. That is, it is primarily designed to explain how competition and monopoly elements work in specific parts of the health care system. This book is not a systematic argument either for more competition or for a different sort of competition.

The Literature

The literature of competition is distributed like that of health economics more generally. Scientific articles can be found in two completely different types of journals. Some can be found in economics journals. More literature is found in health care journals, which are organized by topic, not by discipline. In most such journals, economics articles are rare. But because there are many journals, the total of economics articles in these journals is large. (Only two journals overlap these two categories: the *Journal of Health Economics* and *Health Economics*.)

And yet the journal literature on medical care competition is not the whole of it. Because of intense policy and political interest in health care competition, government reports and court opinions are other im-

1

portant sources of analysis and information.

Research on competition is, by definition, economic research. Yet many who have contributed to the field would not consider themselves economists. Their training might have been in public health, sociology, statistics, health law, health policy, management, nursing, or medicine. These noneconomists, naturally, are especially unlikely to relate their work to the larger body of health economics.

The literature of medical care competition is even more dispersed and less integrated than usual for topics in economics. I hope to impose some unity on an untidy mass of articles, books, papers, and reports.

Organization

Chapter 2 introduces the basic elements of competition in health care. Issues of consumer information and the impact of insurance are first raised here. Unlike the bulk of the book, it does not systematically survey or synthesize the literature. That is left to later chapters on specific parts of the health care industry.

Chapter 3 covers competition among hospitals. Until the mid-1980s, this topic received little attention. But hospitals have been forced to compete more directly, and thus scholarly and policy attention has focused on hospital competition, with a large outpouring of literature in the past few years. Chapter 3 indicates what is known and what is still controversial about hospital competition.

Chapter 4 examines competition among physicians. Unlike the case with hospitals, competition among physicians has long excited policy and scholarly interest. Thus, this chapter includes more historical material and surveys some older material than chapter 3 does, in particular the history of licensure and professional control.

In recent years, the possibility of physician-induced demand has received much attention. This issue is quite distinct analytically from other issues of competition. The literature on supplier-induced demand has developed separately from the other literature on physician competition. For both of these reasons, I have dealt with it separately. Chapter 5 is devoted exclusively to the controversy over physician-induced demand. Some observers believe that such demand is systematically variable and widespread but is not in consumers' interests. This issue probably raises more controversy than any other one analyzed here. This chapter critically surveys the literature. A major goal of this chapter is to explain why statistical studies, even good ones, have not yet resolved the dispute.

Chapter 6 deals with competition among insurers (broadly defined) and how it interacts with competition among doctors and hospitals. Despite the political debate over the performance of private health insurance, the research literature on insurance competition is more unified than might be expected. Among researchers, there is less disagreement about insurance competition than about supplier-induced demand.

In recent years, the theory of adverse selection has been developed and applied to health insurance. Like supply inducement, this area is quite distinct conceptually from the basic literature on insurance competition and thus is treated separately. Chapter 7 presents the basic theory of adverse selection and then examines the use of the term *adverse selection* in policy debates. Finally, related issues of guaranteed insurability and excessive risk sorting are analyzed. Because scholarly or research literature on adverse selection in health insurance or health care is not extensive, this chapter concentrates on independent analysis.

Beyond my conclusions, chapter 8 takes up the issue of whether more competition is, on balance, good or bad, a difficult and debatable topic. After an overview of the issues, the chapter presents my views and points the reader toward the limited literature. A complete discussion of these normative issues is far beyond the scope of this book.

2
Concepts of Competition in Medical Care

At first glance, the American health care industry may appear to be a textbook example of perfect competition. After all, there are many sellers: nationally, there are thousands of hospitals and hundreds of thousands of physicians. Large cities may offer as many as fifty hospitals and thousands of physicians. But competition has been far from perfect. Despite the many sellers, the health care market has not been close to perfectly competitive. Some observers had thought that competition was impossible, unlikely, or even undesirable in health care.

To the surprise of almost everyone, competition in health care has blossomed recently. Health insurance schemes that encourage competition are being introduced. Health maintenance organizations (HMOs) are booming. Preferred provider organizations (PPOs) that negotiate price discounts from providers are growing even faster. Hospitals, especially in California, are making competitive bids for Medicaid and health insurer business. Physicians and hospitals are advertising. Health care marketing specialists, almost nonexistent a decade earlier, are in great demand. This new competition has been subjected to much research, mostly by economists. Often this research sheds light on competitive issues.[1]

But public policy toward health care competition is confused. Federally supported health planning agencies have encouraged hospitals to cooperate to reduce wasteful duplication and to lower costs. But federal antitrust agencies have recently sued hospitals to prevent mergers on standard antitrust grounds. In this book, I hope to present a unified picture of what is known about competition in health care and what is ripe for further research. Through such research, public policy toward competition can be put on a firmer conceptual foundation.

----

1. For generally positive surveys of recent increases in competition, see Paul J. Feldstein (1986), Alain C. Enthoven (1987), and Mark V. Pauly (1988a). For more negative reviews, see Joseph P. Newhouse (1982), Victor R. Fuchs (1986, 1988), and the Congressional Budget Office (1991).

Why Is Competition Imperfect?

Competition in health care is imperfect even where there are many sellers, largely for two reasons. First, consumers are not perfectly informed about the price and quality available from various providers. Second, most health insurance reinforces poor consumer information and undermines the consumer's incentive to use lower-priced providers.

Consumer Information and Monopolistic Competition. Poor consumer information creates many problems in health care. In some cases, a well-informed consumer can treat himself inexpensively, while an ill-informed one must incur costs in seeing a physician. In other cases, a well-informed consumer seeks out a physician, while an ill-informed one does not. Poor information affects what health care is sought and provided. Poor information also reduces competition among providers, the main information problem addressed here. Health care consumers are generally not well informed about their market alternatives. They do not know much about the quality, amenities, or prices for many physicians or hospitals. Further, given traditional health insurance, they may be unwilling to act on information they do have.

As an immediate consequence, each physician is less restrained by competitors than otherwise. Competitors may supply similar services that could easily be substituted. But poor information often causes consumers to view the services of competing providers as different. Poor information exaggerates product differentiation or heterogeneity in the minds of the consumers. Thus, the demand facing physicians is not as elastic as it would be with good information (Nelson 1970). Along a more elastic demand curve, the quantity demanded is more price sensitive.[2]

Individual physicians face downward sloping demand curves. A

---

2. An elasticity gives a measure of the influence—independent of units—of one variable on another. The own-price elasticity of demand, for example, gives the sensitivity of the quantity demanded of a good to its own price. This elasticity is the same whether price is measured in dollars or cents or whether quantity is measured in hundreds or thousands. Algebraically,

$$\text{price elasticity} = \frac{dq}{dp} \cdot \frac{p}{q}, \tag{2-1}$$

where q = quantity, p = price, and dp/dq = the inverse of the slope of the demand curve. Elasticities can be rearranged to be expressed in percentage terms:

physician can raise prices considerably above the competitive level (where price equals marginal cost) without losing all or perhaps even most customers. The higher prices cause patients who stay with the physician to demand less, but they do not spur much switching of physicians. Cross-elasticities of demand among physicians would be lower with poorer information. In other words, with poorer information, the demand for an individual physician would respond less to the prices charged by rivals. Physicians can price more like isolated monopolists. If consumers were perfectly informed, physicians would be more restrained in their price and quality decisions by the fear of losing customers to competitors. The best term to describe the situation is *monopolistic competition*. Though it was once common, explicit collusion among physicians is now rare.

Economists normally use the monopolistically competitive model to describe and to analyze market behavior in health care, especially for physician services (Frech and Ginsburg 1975, 1978; Pauly and Satterthwaite 1981; Satterthwaite 1985; Dranove and Satterthwaite 1991; Zuckerman and Holahan 1991; Pauly 1991; Phelps 1992, 195–201).

For hospitals the situation is similar, although the informational problem is not so acute. For one thing, physicians act as agents for their patients in helping them to select a hospital. Since there are many fewer hospitals than physicians, consumers and their friends and relatives are more likely to have had experience with different hospitals. Hospitals have more brand-name capital than individual practitioners. Conversely, incentives for price search and selection of low-priced hospitals are worse than for selection of low-priced physicians because hospital insurance coverage is more complete than insurance for physician services.

Consumer information will always be costly and imperfect in this market because of the nature of the services. Health insurance, the

---

$$\text{price elasticity} = \frac{\%dq}{\%dp}. \qquad (2\text{--}2)$$

The cross-elasticity of demand (sometimes called the cross-price elasticity) measures the sensitivity of the demand for one good to the price of another good. If the two goods are sold in competition by different sellers, the cross-elasticity of demand measures how closely two sellers compete. Algebraically,

$$\text{cross-elasticity} = \frac{dq_i}{dp_j} \cdot \frac{p_j}{q_i}, \qquad (2\text{--}3)$$

where the i and j subscripts correspond to different sellers. The lower the value of this number, the less directly the two sellers compete.

medical profession, and counterproductive regulation exacerbate the problem. As in many other industries, health care regulation often seems to protect the providers from competition (Olson 1981a, b, 1985; Benham 1978; Benham and Benham 1975; Feldman and Begun 1978).

Poor consumer information may seem an insurmountable barrier to competition. Yet, the market has developed institutions to provide some necessary information, particularly through large group-practices, PPOs, and HMOs. These organizations develop reputations (brand-name capital) over their lives. Further, consumers rely partly on recommendations from a network of friends and relatives in choosing providers. This, in effect, expands the amount of information that they have. Competition through reputation can lead to reasonably efficient markets. And competition does not require that all consumers be well informed. If some consumers are informed well enough to discipline sellers, then competition can work reasonably well.

Perhaps most important, competition is not an absolute; it is a matter of degree. Imperfect information simply means that perfect competition is not attainable. Providers will not act as price takers, as they do in economists' simplified competitive model. Still, the degree of competition is important. In any policy toward competition, it is important not to let the great be the enemy of the good. A small change improving competition is not to be scorned simply because it is a small change.

Just as competition is not an absolute, neither is government regulation, planning, or provision. Even in the most centralized governmental system, different governmental agencies will inevitably compete in the supply of health care. Whether such competition is beneficial depends on exactly how the incentives for consumers and providers are structured. When properly structured, more competition is helpful in many parts of the health care system.

How Monopolistic Competition Works. As the name implies, monopolistic competition has features of both monopoly and competition. The monopoly aspect allows providers to set prices above the competitive level, as described above.

The two competitive aspects apply more easily to physicians than to hospitals. First, providers do not need to consider the reactions of other individual sellers. There are enough closely competitive sellers that providers can simply take their competitors' prices as a given.[3]

---

3. This assumption might not be accurate for hospitals in small markets or for physicians in small specialties. In these cases of small numbers of sellers, direct strategic interactions may play a greater role.

Second, there is mobility among specialties and geographic regions. In the long run, physician mobility will roughly equalize the incomes of (equal quality) physicians across different specialties and areas.[4] But physician mobility will not equalize the relationship of price to cost. The degree of market power can permanently vary across specialties and geographic areas. If so, mobility can equalize only income (more precisely, utility), not the degree of monopoly pricing.

Consumer information and choice as values. Improved consumer information is important for improving competition. As competition improves, health care becomes more efficient. It can lower costs and prices. Or, especially for hospitals, it can lead to higher quality and possibly higher prices. Better information more directly benefits improvement in the choice of the best medical care for each case. Contrary to expectations, this is rarely a technical medical decision. People are not machines waiting to be repaired. The individual values, tastes, limitations, and lifestyles of patients and their families should be considered. The consumer has this information; the physician does not. The consumer's knowledge has become more important because medicine increasingly supplies the subjective benefits of symptomatic relief and comfort. In Victor R. Fuchs's language, "caring" is becoming more important, "curing" less important (1974). Rational medical care requires active consumer choice.

Coronary artery bypass graft (CABG) surgery is a good example of the importance of consumer choice. For about 10 percent of patients, this procedure distinctly improves life expectancy. For another 30 percent, it improves expectancy slightly. But, for fully 60 percent, the procedure does not improve life expectancy at all (Aaron and Schwartz 1984, 64). In the United States, the procedure cost $10,000–25,000 per patient in 1981, for a total cost of $2.5–3.0 billion in that year (Aaron and Schwartz, 63). In most cases, an expensive and somewhat risky procedure is performed solely to reduce chest pain. A correct decision depends on the individual's tolerance for pain, degree of risk aversion, the value placed on other uses of income, and lifestyle.

Though physician advice and attitudes are important, a technocratic medical decision on the bypass operation would be inappropriate. Most relevant information is subjective. Improving consumer information gives a direct benefit in tailoring therapy more accurately

---

4. Income is not perfectly equalized because there are some geographic and specialty barriers to entry and because income is only a rough proxy for utility. Some areas and specialties that are unattractive for personal reasons, for example, must pay higher incomes to attract physicians.

to individuals, as well as sharpening the incentives for competition.

Further, the informational problems that make competition imperfect hinder any effort to replace competition and consumer choice with centralized health care supply or regulation. Central planners are likely to have even more difficulty than consumers in discovering and rewarding the better providers. Planners would be still more disadvantaged deciding how to ration medical care. The informational problems in the medical care system are so great that many decisions must be effectively decentralized. No central planner could decide which individuals get which medical procedure. This key allocative decision must be decentralized. The policy issues concern information flows and incentives. Central planners cannot allocate resources patient by patient.

Excessive Coverage. Health insurance has grown greatly. Both the percentage of consumers with any coverage and the extent of insurance (including employer self-insurance) have grown during the mid- and late twentieth century. The average percentage of health care bills paid by public or private health care insurers rose from about 12 percent to about 78 percent from 1929 to 1991, with the most rapid growth complete before 1970. By eradicating the financial risk of large medical bills for many people, insurance has been a blessing to American consumers. But health insurance has negative side effects.

The large subsidy of health care has markedly increased health care expenditures. These greater expenditures reflect partly more income and partly improved medical technology. They also result from the growth in insurance. Some of this growth is a necessary byproduct of any insurance. But insurance, at least for the middle class, is overly complete. That is, its copayments are insufficient, and its utilization review is not aggressive enough. This insurance has caused more inefficiency than necessary.

Moral hazard. By reducing the effective or out-of-pocket price of health care, insurance raises demand. This is called moral hazard. The concept was brought into economics from the insurance industry by Mark V. Pauly (1968). The term applies to the situation where the incentives created by the insurance induce the policyholders to change their behavior so that losses to consumers increase. In the insurance industry, the term *moral hazard* was applied to such acts as arson. Not surprisingly, insurers considered this immoral behavior. The connotation of immorality may seem a bit out of place in health insurance, but the colorful language of moral hazard has stuck.

According to extensive research, utilization and expenditures are higher for more completely insured consumers. The most reliable study (Newhouse et al. 1981; Manning et al. 1987; Newhouse et al. 1993) showed that moving from a fairly large deductible (about $1,000 per family in 1977) to complete (100 percent, first-dollar) insurance raised expenditures about 50 percent. Moral hazard applies to both the quantity and the quality dimensions of the choice of health care. Unless quantity and quality are strongly substitutable (which seems impossible), more insurance coverage will cause consumers to demand both more health care and better care than otherwise. But more is known about how moral hazard increases utilization than about how it raises the quality and cost per unit of health care.

Optimal insurance. There is a trade-off between spreading risk and moral hazard. More insurance causes more moral hazard, hence more waste. But more insurance reduces financial risk. Either too little or too much insurance is wasteful. Optimal insurance balances the two effects. The marginal benefit from spreading risk is equal to the marginal loss from moral hazard. Optimal insurance always covers less than 100 percent of losses.[5]

Many economists believe that, on average, Americans have too much health insurance. Health insurance payments are tax deductible to employers and employees. This subsidizes the purchase of excessively complete group health insurance (Feldstein and Friedman 1977; Pauly 1980a, 1986, 1987a; Congressional Budget Office 1994). This subsidy does not promote health insurance for the poor, the unemployed, or the self-employed. Further, the Blue Cross/Blue Shield plans use their market power to promote more complete insurance (Frech 1974, 1979, 1980a; Frech and Ginsburg 1978a, 1981, 1988; Hay and Leahy 1984; Pauly 1988c).

While those with group insurance are likely to be overinsured, many consumers have no insurance. Willard G. Manning and M. Susan Marquis (1989) conclude that in the aggregate there is too much insurance and it is maldistributed. Optimality requires less insurance for most of the middle class with group insurance and more insurance for the (largely lower income) people with little or no insurance.

The literature contains many estimates of the welfare loss of the

---

5. There are other adverse effects of more complete insurance. Optimal insurance is less complete than what would be suggested by the simple trade-off of moral hazard versus risk spreading that is featured in the literature. Several writers have shown that in a competitive and unsubsidized market with unavoidable moral hazard, consumers would choose such optimally incomplete insurance (Zeckhauser 1970; Frech 1974, 1979; and Pauly 1974a, 1980a, 1986).

excessive health insurance (Feldstein 1973; Manning et al. 1987; Manning and Marquis 1989; Feldman and Dowd 1991). But this literature considers additional moral hazard as the only cost of more complete insurance. By ignoring the effect of insurance on reducing competition, this literature understates the economic harm of excessive insurance.

Insurance and health care competition. Health insurance of the traditional hands-off, third-party type reduces competition. This effect is more subtle than a simple slide down a demand curve, but it is no less important. Different types of insurance have different effects. The most common type of insurance reduces the incentives for consumers to search for lower prices. It reduces the willingness of consumers to patronize the lower-priced physicians or hospitals. Therefore, it gives providers more market power.

The rational consumer searches up to the point where the expected gain of further search equals the cost. Consider the gains to search. Without insurance or any other subsidy, the consumer keeps all the savings from searching out a lower price. If he were looking for an automobile, for example, and he found a lower price at a more distant dealer, he would pocket the entire price difference. The situation is entirely different for the consumer with the typical type of health insurance.

The worst case is complete insurance with no copayment at all. Although this kind of coverage is becoming less popular, it is still used by Medicaid; Medicare uses a version for hospital insurance (there is a copayment, but it does not vary by hospital). Complete insurance is also still used by Blue Cross/Blue Shield plans, especially where they have large market shares. Some commercial insurance covers 100 percent, but it is becoming rare.

Insurance also reduces the cost of search to the extent that a search takes the form of consuming medical care. Much health care consumer search takes place by obtaining recommendations from friends and relatives; this activity is not subsidized by insurance. Often, sampling medical care is impossible: a consumer can receive only one appendectomy. Even when sampling medical care is possible, only the direct monetary cost of the care is subsidized, not the transportation or time. Thus, insurance will reduce search.

Consumers with this 100 percent insurance coverage have no incentive at all to become informed about lower-priced sources of health care. Even if they did somehow become informed, they have no incentive to choose such providers. They will simply choose the provider that they most prefer with cost as no object. It does not matter whether the same care could be obtained at a much lower cost elsewhere. If

11

there were even a slight disadvantage to the lower-priced provider, the consumer would not change. For these consumers, there can be no price competition at all. Such an insurance scheme cannot become the norm without destroying the market.

If all consumers were 100 percent insured, provider pricing would not be constrained. A higher price would not discourage consumers at all. Conversely, a lower price would not attract them. Price competition would become completely futile. Since providers had profits to gain by raising prices and nothing to lose, prices would rise without limit. H. E. Frech and Paul Ginsburg (1975, 1978b) have called this the explosive case. Such a price explosion has not happened and is not happening. The price system is being maintained largely by consumers who have either incomplete insurance or none at all.[6] These are the consumers who have some price sensitivity and some incentive to search for and choose lower-cost sellers. Those with 100 percent coverage are free riding on the search and choice efforts of other consumers.

Coinsurance. Coinsurance is the percentage of the bill that the consumer must pay out-of-pocket, commonly 20 percent. Those who pay coinsurance have some incentive for search and choice of price-competitive providers because they keep 20 percent of the savings. Though they have attenuated incentives, these consumers are important to competition because of their numbers. This is probably the largest group of privately insured consumers. It includes most of those with commercial insurance, some with Blue Cross/Blue Shield insurance and some with Medicare insurance for physicians. These consumers benefit when they discover and choose a lower-priced provider, but not to the full extent of the savings that they uncover. They must share the savings with the insurance company, according to the sharing rule implied by their coinsurance.

Suppose such a consumer's physician charged $200 for a particular procedure. If the consumer found another physician who charged only $100, he would save by switching. But the extent of his saving would be reduced by the coinsurance. If the coinsurance rate were 20 percent, he would save himself $20 but would save the insurance company more, $80. The expected value of search to the consumer is only 20 percent of what it would have been if he had been uninsured. Thus, he would stop searching sooner and make his choice with poorer information. If he were satisfied with his current provider, he might not search at all. Further, even if he knew about the lower-priced provider, often he would not use it.

---

6. There is also some restraint by the formal and informal rules used by insurers to limit their payment to "reasonable" prices.

If it were worth $21 more to the consumer to use the high-priced provider (perhaps because of a more convenient location), he would use him. The consumer gains services worth $21 to himself by so doing, but the services cost $100 more to produce.

Deductibles. Deductibles are more complicated than coinsurance. For our purposes, it is enough to say that they work like coinsurance, where the probability that the deductible will be exceeded plays a role similar to that of coinsurance. That is, the higher the probability of exceeding the deductible, the less concerned about price and cost the consumer is (Keeler, Newhouse, and Phelps 1973). Therefore, deductibles do not improve search or incentives for services whose costs are sure to exceed them, such as open heart surgery.

It may seem that insurance would suppress searching for lower prices but not for quality information. This is not necessarily so. Less price search might imply less search on the nature of the services as well.

Indemnity insurance. Coinsurance and deductibles are not the only ways to improve consumer search and utilization incentives. Indemnity insurance is another approach that offers the possibility of combining insurance with far better incentives than coinsurance. The term *indemnity* is used to mean at least three different things (Pauly 1986). One is simply a payment defined in money terms rather than a promise to provide services. A distinction without a difference, this is sometimes said to distinguish Blue Cross/Blue Shield plans from the commercial insurers.[7] The second meaning is an insurance benefit that pays a certain amount depending on the state of the world—here the onset of illness—whether or not the consumer uses any medical care. Indemnities of this sort are rare in health insurance, typically limited to easily observable and measurable injuries. Accidental dismemberment policies, for example, might pay $10,000 for the loss of a leg.

Finally, I use the term *indemnity* to denote insurance that provides coverage up to a fixed dollar amount per unit of service provided. It may, for example, provide $25,000 per coronary bypass operation, $50 per physician visit, or $500 per hospital day. This type of insurance is more common than is generally believed. Many commercial policies

---

7. Service benefits plans are sometimes said to be those where the provider handles the paperwork and does not charge the patient any balance bills. This description, however, fits some commercial plans, especially PPOs. Also, some Blue Cross/Blue Shield plans allow balance billing by member physicians. And most of them allow consumers to choose nonmember providers, who may not handle the paperwork and who can balance bill.

and some Blue Cross/Blue Shield policies are explicitly called indemnity benefits, especially for physician services. But payment limits in coinsured and full-coverage policies convert them to, in effect, indemnity policies.

Consider the case of price limits, called allowances, common to most Blue Shield or commercial benefits and to all Medicare physician services benefits. In all states, except Massachusetts, consumers can patronize physicians who charge more than the Blue Shield or Medicare allowance. This practice, called balance billing, converts the policy into an indemnity policy, with the indemnity payment equal to the percentage paid by the insurer times the allowed price.

Thus, Medicare provides, in effect, indemnity insurance for physician services where the indemnity amount is 80 percent of the Medicare allowance. About one-fifth of Medicare physician services charges are balance billed.[8] The possibility of balance billing encourages consumers to search for physicians who do not balance bill (called accepting assignment in Medicare jargon). For physician services, the original Medicare benefit design was reasonably efficient and procompetitive. Most physicians who do not balance bill Medicare enrollees reduce their prices to do so. Private insurance that supplements Medicare, called Medigap insurance, often fills in the coinsurance and sometimes the balance bills and thus undermines the incentives.

Coinsurance benefits are converted into indemnity in yet another way. Some physicians and some dentists waive the coinsurance, in full or in part. If they waive the entire coinsurance, they offer to accept a percentage of the insurer's allowance as payment in full. The provider generally grants a discount to the consumer below his usual fees to do this. This form of competitive price cutting is more effective than simply cutting one's regular fees. If a provider were to cut his regular fees, the bulk of the price reduction would benefit the insurer, not the consumer. Thus, it would be less effective in attracting consumers than waiving the coinsurance would be.

Twenty-three percent of privately insured consumers report having coinsurance waived at least once in the past three years (Lachs, Sindelar, and Horowitz 1990).

The practice of waiving the coinsurance in effect converts the coinsured service benefits into indemnity insurance. This encourages competition among providers. Indeed, waiving the coinsurance is itself largely an attempt to compete more effectively on the basis of prices. Some insurers, especially those controlled by providers, such as the

---

8. An unknown percentage of physicians do not accept assignment but do not attempt to collect the balance bills from their Medicare customers.

California Dental Service (also called California Delta Dental), oppose these practices.

The difference in attitude between ordinary insurers and those controlled by providers is easy to explain. By stopping providers from waiving the coinsurance, the provider-controlled insurers discourage competition among their membership. This is in the interests of the provider-members who control these insurers. Ordinary commercial insurers, conversely, would prefer more competition among the providers serving their customers.[9]

Indemnity insurance leaves the incentives for the search and choice of lower-priced providers almost unaltered from the uninsured situation. Indemnity insurance makes the consumer the residual payer if the indemnity benefit level is set below the prices of most providers. Consider the consumer choice, discussed above, between a physician charging $100 and one charging $200. If the indemnity plan were to pay $90, the consumer's incentives to search and to choose the lower-priced physician would be strong, the same as if he were completely uninsured. If the consumer chose the lower-priced physician, his out-of-pocket expense would be $10, while if he chose the higher-priced one, his out-of-pocket payment would be $110. The difference, the cost saving, would be $100. The consumer would not share this with the insurer. Thus, he would extend his search further and more likely would choose the lower-priced provider. Thus, economists have often recommended indemnity features for efficient insurance (Frech and Ginsburg 1975, 1978b; Pauly 1971b, 1986; Newhouse and Taylor 1970, 1971).

Consumers with indemnity insurance are more likely to become informed of price differences and change their choices in response to price changes. From the viewpoint of the provider, the incentive to price more competitively is stronger. The provider would find that he lost more patients in response to a price rise than if his patients had coinsurance. Indemnity insurance, therefore, promotes competition.[10]

Until about 1975, health insurance was becoming progressively

---

9. For an alternative viewpoint on waiving the coinsurance that stresses charitable and fraudulent motives, rather than competitive ones, see Mark S. Lachs, Jody L. Sindelar, and Ralph I. Horowitz (1990).

10. Indemnity insurance has another advantage over coinsurance. It shifts the demand curve upward parallel to the original (by the amount of the indemnity benefit). Coinsurance rotates the demand curve around its intercept with the quantity axis. Even if providers were perfect monopolists, indemnity insurance would constrain their monopolistic pricing with a more elastic demand curve than coinsurance (Frech and Ginsburg 1975, 1978b).

more complete, and indemnity features were becoming less common. There has been a dramatic change since then. Deductibles and coinsurance are increasing. Indemnity features are increasing. Also, PPOs are flourishing. These insurance reforms are contributing to better-informed consumers and therefore causing the health care market to become more competitive.

Levels of Competition

There are two distinct levels of competition in health care. Both are attenuated, when compared with the typical manufacturing industry. One is competition to enter the market. For physicians, this is limited by licensure and the control of medical education (Kessel 1958; Frech 1975; Leffler 1978; Leffler and Lindsay 1981). For hospitals, entry is constrained by the necessity of accreditation by the American Hospital Association to receive payment from many governmental programs. At the state level, licensure is an impediment, but state licensure requirements are not generally stringent. Local cartels and collusions sometimes limit hospital entry (Shalit 1977; Frech 1979). Historically, the local hospital planning associations tried to discourage entry and expansion by voluntary methods, with varying success (Grosse 1974). In the 1970s, certificate-of-need (CON) laws were passed by most states and written into the Medicare law. The CON laws, common in the 1970s, required a planning agency to approve entry or expansion.

Partly because of research discussed later in this book, these laws and the health planning movement behind them have fallen into disrepute. The federal government has withdrawn funding from such planning agencies. And many states have repealed or weakened their CON laws. In that spirit, the following chapters do not focus on entry limitation, but concentrate more on the issue of competition among those physicians or hospitals that have already entered the market.

3
Competition among Hospitals

Public policy toward hospital competition has zigzagged between two contradictory paths. An older tradition of local health and hospital planning and regulation, which perhaps peaked in the late 1960s, still influences policy. It favors hospital cooperation, or collusion, either through the local planning process or independent of it. The planning tradition also favors hospital mergers, in part because they reduce competition (Grosse 1974, 28). Passage of the National Health Planning and Resources Development Act of 1974 reflected this generally anti-competitive view. The law was an attempt to supplement or to replace market forces, and especially competition, with local planning. In the early, optimistic days of health planning, Congress appeared to believe that hospital mergers that violated the antitrust laws could be socially beneficial (Miles 1984).

The failure of planning and regulation to control costs has renewed interest in competition as a cost-control policy. Because research and research funding in health economics are sensitive to policy interests, the change in perspectives has spawned new research on hospital competition. As faith in regulation and planning faded with experience, antitrust enforcement officials have taken more initiatives in health policy. Prompted by this major intellectual and policy movement beginning in the early 1970s, the Federal Trade Commission (FTC) and the Department of Justice have challenged hospital mergers, with a traditional antitrust view (*American Medical International* 1984). These policies have continued, regardless of the political party in power.

Market Developments. Simultaneously, rapid changes in health insurance have made the health care market more competitive. Managed insurance plans such as HMOs and PPOs have flourished. These plans aid the consumer by acting as an informed purchasing agent in selecting price-competitive hospitals. Consumer copayments are becoming more common. Higher copayments induce the consumer to be more sensitive to price. The procompetitive insurance developments have also spurred research on hospital competition.

17

New Research. Both the policy interest and the market developments in health insurance have stimulated a wave of new research on the nature of hospital competition. The new work is mostly empirical and focuses on the effect of concentration or the number of competitors on various measures of hospital output. Much of the older line of research, primarily on collusion to limit entry, is really an extension of the analysis of physician competition.

Entry Limitation

The Hospital Planning Movement. Just as for physicians, entry limitation has been important for hospital care. Though the details are obscure, the main mechanisms of entry limitation are clear enough. In many locales, existing hospitals have long cooperated through formal or informal local hospital planning agencies or committees (Grosse 1974). These groups were influenced by physicians, the hospitals themselves, and major donors. Without their approval, new nonprofit hospitals experienced fund-raising difficulties in entering the market. The same was true for an expansion of an existing hospital. These planning groups generally opposed entry by profit-seeking hospitals and by HMOs.

Such groups had a clear and sophisticated rationale for their actions. Because of the moral hazard effect of hospital insurance, consumers demand too much hospital care of too high a quality. To curtail that situation, one could simply limit the supply of hospital care through direct controls on entry and expansion. Clearly, limiting competition served the interests of the hospitals. What motivated the donors is less clear; most likely, they believed the rationale of the planning movement.

Local Physician Cartels. The relationship of the planning movement to physicians' interest is fascinating. Sol Shalit (1977) has shown theoretically that a doctors' cartel would favor restrictions on the supply of complementary hospital services since this would reduce the supply of physician services and raise prices: states and urban areas with fewer hospital beds per capita have higher hospital and physician prices.

Other research supports these findings. Frech (1979) showed that, with length of stay constant, daily hospital costs and daily room charges were lower in states where hospital beds were plentiful. Costs per admission would also be lower. Pauly (1980b) and Frank A. Sloan (1982) found that physician prices were higher where hospital beds were more scarce and where hospitals had fewer nursing services. William S. Custer (1986) reported that where hospitals were more competitive, physician prices were lower. Further, Frech (1979) found that the quantity of hospital beds or bed days supplied was almost independent of the price. This suggests that the varying strength of the local hospital or physician cartels determines hospital supply, not the usual economic factors. (These studies were based on data before the enactment of formal governmental restrictions on entry.)

Certificate-of-Need Regulation. In considering hospital entry-limiting regulation from the aspect of public choice or political economy, Shalit defines organized medicine broadly and includes hospital associations. He found that organized medicine has always favored restricting hospital supply, but this is overbroad. Paul J. Feldstein (1977) pointed out major differences in the political and policy positions of the various health provider organizations. He stressed that the American Medical Association (AMA) has long opposed certificate-of-need (CON) (see chapter 2) regulation and supported the Hill-Burton program that subsidized rural hospitals. Additional research on the political economy of hospital limitation would be valuable.

In any case, by 1974 several states had instituted CON laws. In that year, Congress mandated the laws for the rest of the states (Gelman 1982, 4). Most research shows that this regulation had little or no effect on hospital costs (Sloan and Steinwald 1980; Sloan 1981; Misek and Reynolds 1982; and Anderson 1991).[1] If the studies had included the increased prices for physician services, the results of regulation would have looked even worse.

The higher hospital costs represent a gain to those controlling the hospitals, whether physicians or not. The higher demand for each bed allows the hospitals to pursue costly technology, interesting cases, managerial slack, and so on. Supply reduction leads to higher quality in the eyes of hospital decision makers. But consumers are unlikely to believe that the improvement is worth the higher cost. Otherwise, it would have been chosen in competitive markets. Some of the higher quality is probably detrimental. The often-criticized excessively technical nature of U.S. medical care is partly due to hospital market power, unwittingly amplified by entry-limiting regulation.

CON regulation has also inhibited competition from HMOs by

---

1. Two exceptions are the studies of John Mayo and Deborah McFarland (1989, 1991). They claim that CON regulation has reduced both the number of beds and total costs in Tennessee. Keith Anderson (1991) points out some econometric problems with their work. The most serious seems to be their use of the percentage of CON applications turned down as their measure of CON strictness. This variable seems to be endogenous.

stopping them from building hospitals. Doctors and existing hospitals in the San Fernando Valley of Los Angeles, for example, used certificate-of-need to delay Kaiser's second hospital for years (Manning 1990).

Partly because of the research by Sloan and others, hospital certificate-of-need regulation has lost its appeal. Under more permissive federal legislation, many states have quietly dropped this form of regulation (Ryon 1984). But the recent trend of fewer hospital admissions and shorter stays may have made both the cartel and the regulatory restraints on entry irrelevant.

The Nonprofit Nature of Hospitals

Most U.S. hospitals are private, nonprofit corporations. Of the remainder, about half are government owned, most by local governments. Nonprofit firms of both types might be expected to behave differently from profit-seeking ones. According to the property rights theory of the firm (Alchian 1961; Williamson 1970; Alchian and Demsetz 1972), the nonprofit status adds constraints to a firm. These constraints affect the trade-off between pecuniary and nonpecuniary benefits made by the top decision makers. A nonprofit firm cannot pay dividends. Therefore, the nonprofit constraint allows the top decision makers to pursue nonpecuniary goals with less or even no cost to themselves but with additional costs to the firm.[2] The literature suggests several goals for hospitals, including prestige, quantity and quality of care, charity care, research, administrative slack, and physician income (Sloan 1988; Hoerger 1991). Hoerger provided indirect evidence that nonprofit hospitals do allow greater administrative slack.

The various nonprofit models differ from each other and from the simple profit-maximizing model in their predictions regarding the levels of variables. They predict, for example, different outcomes for prices, costs, type of services provided, and quality and quantity of services for hospitals facing identical demand and cost conditions. In particular, most models predict that nonprofit hospitals would set prices lower than profit-seeking hospitals. The empirical evidence con-

---

2. Many studies focus on the differences in efficiency between private property (profit-seeking) firms and nonprofit or governmental ones. The researchers had to deal with the problem that nonprofit firms often produce output of subtly different quality or type. Most, though not all, studies found that private property firms had lower costs. This approach has been applied to nursing homes (Borjas, Frech, and Ginsburg 1983; Frech 1985; Weisbrod and Schlesinger 1983) and to health insurers (Frech 1976; Vogel and Blair 1975a, 1975b).

firms this: nonprofit hospitals set prices about 10 to 15 percent lower for the same type of care (Sloan 1988; Noether 1986; Woolley 1987). Conversely, in other measurable ways, even in costs and in the extent of charity care, profit-seeking and nonprofit hospitals are similar (Sloan 1988). For theoretical reasons, one would expect them to be similar in how they respond to changes in their economic environment.

Response to Change. Comparative statics is the study of how the behavior of a firm or market responds to changes in its environment; the static equilibriums before and after a change are compared. The comparative statics of profit-seeking and nonprofit hospitals are likely to be similar.

To understand this, we should think of those who control nonprofit hospitals as making their decisions in two steps. First, they maximize profits. Second, since they cannot keep the profits, they spend them on nonpecuniary goals by reducing prices, adding equipment and services, reducing management effort, and so on. Now consider a change; perhaps the demand curve facing the hospital becomes more price elastic because a new PPO is formed. The hospital cannot operate as it as before. Whatever the ultimate nonpecuniary goods its decision makers favor, the hospital must respond to the demand change by reducing its price and its implicit profits. At its new optimum in the more competitive world, the nonprofit hospital charges a lower price. This is the same direction of response to the change that a profit-maximizing hospital would make. Pauly (1974; 1987b) and Dranove, Satterthwaite, and Sindelar (1986, 428) argued that both theoretical and empirical analysis suggests similar behavior for profit-seeking and nonprofit hospitals.[3] Thus, many policies affect profit-seeking and nonprofit hospitals in roughly the same way.

Nonprofit Hospital Collusion. Further, the nonprofit hospital, just like its profit-seeking counterpart, has incentives to collude with its competitors. Nonprofit hospitals are probably more likely to collude than profit-seeking ones. First, nonprofit hospitals have a tradition of collusion with each other and with major donors that dates back at least to the days of voluntary hospital planning. Further, the decision makers of nonprofit hospitals are likely to have similar values, including cooperation. Nonprofit hospitals are more likely than profit-seeking ones to be dominated by their medical staffs, many of whom are also on the

---

3. For a contrary view (that nonprofit hospitals are less likely to charge higher prices in concentrated markets), see William Lynk (1995).

staffs of competing hospitals (Clark 1980; Bays 1983; Sloan 1988). This overlap of medical staff facilitates hospital collusion.

Cream Skimming. The decision makers of nonprofit hospitals are also likely to place a similar value on which services to overprice and which ones to subsidize. Jeffrey Harris (1979, 233) found strong similarities in the pricing of a sample of nonprofit hospitals. Generally, large monopoly rents were earned on routine ancillary services such as X-rays and on daily room charges, while surgical support services were underpriced. Harris argues that this pattern of monopoly pricing is consistent with charitable motivation and economic efficiency. On the contrary, Carson Bays (1983, 370–73) believes that physicians have traditionally favored nonprofit hospitals because physicians can control them more easily. He also believes that the cross-subsidy favoring surgery simply reflects the economic interest of surgeons and harms the poor. Conversely, nonprofit hospital subsidies for maternity care and emergency rooms probably favor the poor.

Profit-seeking hospitals are often accused of cream skimming—undercutting the nonprofit hospitals' highest prices. This is natural. Competition is attracted first to the services that are the most overpriced. The accusation reflects the fact that profit-seeking hospitals are less likely to follow the explicit collusion or implicit communality of interests of the nonprofit hospitals. As mavericks or spoilers, profit-seeking hospitals would be expected to inject more competition into their markets.

One would expect the same response by nonprofit and profit-seeking hospitals to changes in the economic environment. Therefore, most literature on hospital competition uses the simplifying assumption of profit maximization. Although the presence of profit-seeking hospitals may not affect price changes, it affects the level of prices in two ways. Profit-seeking hospitals charge more. Conversely, their more aggressive competition leads to lower prices by their nonprofit competitors. Empirical work usually allows the presence of profit-seeking hospitals to affect the level of prices.

Competition among Existing Hospitals

Because of the informational and incentive problems discussed above, hospital competition is imperfect, even in cities with many alternatives within a short distance. Further, there are many markets with just a few competing hospitals so that oligopolistic interactions further reduce effective competition.

Collusion. Because of a long history of collusion and cooperation among hospitals, partly nurtured by local hospital planning agencies, direct collusion is common. The planners in Delaware, for example, brag that the state's low hospital-bed-to-population ratio "has been achieved through the voluntary cooperation and joint planning efforts among Delaware hospitals" (*Health Plan for Delaware* 1984, 339).

Collusion among hospitals typically focuses on easily observable elements of nonprice competition, such as the number of beds or the services offered. Price collusion would be difficult to enforce because of the complexity of the bundle of services that constitute hospital care (Woolley and Frech 1988–89). In 1975, for example, the three Modesto, California, hospitals agreed to allocate several services among themselves. The services assigned by agreement included prenatal care, radiation therapy, computerized automated tomography scanning, and renal dialysis (Woolley and Frech 1988–89, 63).

The Existence of Competition

Much evidence refutes the monopoly model of the hospital market. But before we consider this, we need to be precise about how we use the terms *competition* and *monopoly*. I use the standard economic definitions, which differ a bit from both the legal and the vernacular definitions.

Monopoly means that each independent hospital can raise its prices without fear of losing any patients to other hospitals. Each potential patient will demand less; some patients may decide not to use the hospital at all; but none will switch to other hospitals. In technical terms cross-elasticities of demand among hospitals are zero.[4] In this situation, each hospital faces a demand curve that is simply a portion of the total market demand curve. Each hospital is completely isolated economically in the output market. (Hospitals may compete for inputs, such as nurses.) Alternatively, the same result would occur if all the hospitals colluded perfectly.

Competition is the opposite extreme. Under perfect competition, each hospital is a price taker. It can sell all the services it wants at the going price and nothing at all at a price even slightly higher than this.

Market Demand Is Too Inelastic for Monopoly. If the market were perfectly monopolistic, each hospital would face a demand curve that was just a miniature version of the market demand curve. In particular,

---

4. The cross-elasticity of demand measures how sensitive the demand for one seller is to the price of a possible competitor. See above footnote 3 of chapter 2 for a formal definition.

23

it would have the same price elasticity of demand.

Individual hospitals can increase total revenue, thus profits, by raising prices if the demand curve facing them is price-inelastic (elasticity of demand less than 1.0 in absolute value).[5] If the demand is inelastic, a price increase raises total revenue while reducing the quantity supplied (and therefore total costs). Thus, one will never observe a profit-maximizing firm selling where its own individual demand curve is inelastic. If a firm finds itself in this position, it will raise its price well into the elastic region of its demand curve.

Under the assumption of monopoly, the demand elasticity facing individual hospitals is the same as that facing the industry as a whole. Therefore, both the industry and the firm-level demand curves for hospital care would have to be price-elastic. But study after study shows that the industrywide demand for hospital care is inelastic, around −0.2. Such a finding is incompatible with monopoly.

One may object that hospitals have chosen not to exploit their market power fully, so that the above analysis does not apply. While there is undoubtedly some truth to the idea that some hospitals have not exploited all their monopoly power, many hospitals are failing. If they did not have to compete, these hospitals would face the relatively inelastic market demand curve. If so, they could simply raise their prices, earn more monopoly rents, and prosper.

Further, about 9 percent of hospitals are profit-seeking. Surely the shareholders of these firms hope and believe that these hospitals are using all their monopoly power. There is some evidence, discussed below, that the average profit-seeking hospital charges more than comparable nonprofit firms. The difference is small, perhaps 10 to 15 percent. If the hospitals were truly facing the industry demand curve as required by the pure monopoly model, they would have to raise their prices more than 200 percent to achieve the profit-maximizing price. See appendix 3-A.

Selling below Market Prices. If hospitals were monopolies, they would be under no pressure to grant discounts to small buyers. (Large buyers might be able to depress their prices by their monopsony power.) No buyer would shift to another hospital despite the price difference. Yet, hospitals often grant discounts of 10 to 20 percent to small private PPOs and HMOs (Dranove, Satterthwaite, and Sindelar 1986,

---

5. If quantity supplied decreases, costs decline as well. Thus, a price increase that raised total revenue and reduced quantity would, of necessity, raise profits.

421; Frech 1988b). Thus, hospitals must offer discounts to keep from losing business to competitors.

This pattern of price discounts cannot be explained by monopolistic price discrimination at the individual level. The individual customers of HMOs and PPOs do not have more elastic demand curves for hospital care. The demand curve at the level of the individual hospital is more elastic because of the threat that the HMOs and PPOs will take consumers away if prices are too high. Some may argue that the discounts can also be explained by charitable motivation. This is not true when lower prices are charged for private PPOs and HMOs. Consumers with this type of insurance are not usually poor.

Consumer Choice of Provider and Insurance. The monopoly model also predicts that the provider chosen by consumers will be independent of the price to the consumer. This implies that the provider chosen should also be independent of the type of insurance held. The available evidence shows that consumers with indemnity insurance choose lower-priced physicians and hospitals than those with coinsured benefits (Newhouse and Phelps 1974) and that consumers with more complete Blue Cross hospital insurance choose more costly hospitals (Andersen and Anderson 1970). See the discussion below.

Imperfect Competition

The opposite extreme from the monopoly model is the perfectly competitive model. It is as easy to disprove as the monopoly model is.

Selling below Market Prices. Perfectly competitive hospitals would not sell their services below market prices. They could sell all they wanted at the going, competitive price. Actual hospitals sell some services at a discount. Medicare, Medicaid, some Blue Cross plans, and most HMOs and PPOs receive discounts. The magnitudes vary. Many PPOs get discounts in the 20 percent range. California Medicaid (Medi-Cal) gets about a 12 percent average discount on hospital services by competitive bidding. Despite this, more than 60 percent of California hospitals contract with it (Dranove, Satterthwaite, and Sindelar 1986, 421). Medicaid discounts in Minneapolis are at least 15 percent, yet almost all hospitals have Medicaid patients (Feldman and Dowd 1986, 285). No doubt there is some effort to supply lower-quality services to the discount patients, especially the Medicaid ones. But the ability to reduce quality selectively in a publicly observable setting is severely limited. Moreover, some hospitals try to discourage Medicaid admis-

sions, but the results from the California competitive bidding procedure show that these hospitals are in the minority. Most California
hospitals offered discounts.

The granting of discounts to Medicaid patients is consistent with
a charitable motive, but the granting of discounts to HMOs, PPOs, and
Blue Cross plans is not. These patients have above-average income and
insurance coverage.

Demand Facing Individual Hospitals. As explained above, if hospitals
were monopolists, they would face demand curves with the same elasticity as demand curves the hospital industry faces as a whole, about
-0.2. Perfectly competitive hospitals would face an elasticity of demand of minus infinity. Clearly, the truth is somewhere between these
extremes. There are two methods for estimating this elasticity facing
an individual hospital.

The first method uses the willingness of hospitals to accept discounts for certain patients. For the hospital indifferent whether it
serves some patients at a discount or refuses to serve them, its marginal
cost is equal to the discounted price. Knowing the magnitude of the
discount, we can solve the first-order conditions for profit maximization for the implied elasticity of demand facing the hospital:

$$\text{marginal revenue} = \text{price} \left(1 + \frac{1}{\eta}\right) \qquad (3\text{--}1)$$

where η is the price elasticity of demand facing the individual hospital.

Roger Feldman and Bryan Dowd (1986) applied this technique to
1981 data from Minneapolis–St. Paul hospitals. They distinguished
prices to four different groups: Medicare, Medicaid, Blue Cross, and
all non-Medicare, non-Medicaid (Blue Cross, commercial insurance, including HMOs, self-pay, charity, workmen's compensation). Because
the price of hospital care is complex, they used a hedonic technique to
control for case mix (diagnosis and severity). Not surprisingly, they
found that Medicaid paid the least and Blue Cross paid the most for
hospital care. The implied elasticity of demand facing an individual
hospital for all private (non-Medicare, non-Medicaid) patients was
-3.94 per day and -6.26 for an admission. For Blue Cross patients,
with their more complete insurance, the demand was naturally less
elastic, at -2.31 and -3.69, respectively (1986, 285).

They also directly estimated demand equations at the level of the
individual hospital. These equations related the quantity of hospital
care provided to each payer group to the case mix–adjusted price to
that group and to other variables designed to hold quality constant
(public ownership, existence of a teaching program, and the number

of services available). Here, the estimated price elasticities of demand are significantly lower, -0.744 for private-pay days and -1.124 for Blue Cross admissions (1986, 290). The authors suggest that there is a measurement error in the price for private-pay patients. Some private-pay patients receive discounts, and some do not.

But there are other possible explanations. First, there are other sources of error in the price variable. The hedonic adjustment for case mix, however nicely done, is far from perfect. Perhaps more serious, the quality and amenities vary across hospitals. The higher-quality and amenity hospitals tend to be larger and more expensive. Therefore, the estimated effect of price on quantity will be biased toward zero. This will result in measured price elasticities that understate the true constant-quality ones. This problem recurs in the attempts to estimate physician-level demand curves directly.

The study also showed the importance of nonprice competition. The availability of a wide range of services attracted private patients, as did the presence of a medical teaching program. Public ownership strongly discouraged private patients. Even Medicare patients were responsive to these proxies for quality, though they could not respond to price (since their small copayments are independent of hospital price).

Luft, Garnick, Mark, Peltzman, Phibbs, Lichtenberg, and McPhee (1990) confirmed these results and added some. First, patients were more likely to choose hospitals with good mortality outcomes (even before such data were public), holding constant other observable proxies for quality such as medical school affiliation and size. Further, surgery admissions were both more price sensitive and more quality sensitive than medical admissions. This is consistent with the idea that the market rewards to high quality are highest in the surgical specialties (Dranove and Satterthwaite 1991). It is also consistent with a price discrimination interpretation of hospital cross-subsidies, which usually favor surgery. Further, surgical admissions are more likely to be planned in advance and to require referral from a primary care physician. Both factors make informed choices easier.

In the earlier study, Feldman and Dowd estimated price elasticities of demand for private patients that range from -0.744 to -3.94. These elasticities are small enough (in absolute value) to reject perfect competition, even for urban hospitals. The smallest implied monopolistic markup, for the most elastic estimate, is a substantial 17 percent above marginal costs.

Conversely, the estimates are far more elastic than those for the hospital industry as a whole. This implies that hospitals can shift patients away from their competitors by reducing price. Thus, even urban hospitals have a significant amount of market power, but they are far from monopolists. Clearly, price competition among hospitals exists.

Does Hospital Competition Have Perverse Results?

Because of poor consumer information and high insurance coverage, the effect of hospital competition on efficiency and consumer welfare is unclear. The traditional antitrust approach suggests that hospital competition would reduce the price of a constant-quality hospital day and make the system more responsive to consumers.

But some writers have argued that competition among hospitals increases costs and prices. Excessive nonprice competition leads to overuse of technology and other resources. Normal price-reducing market pressures are believed to be absent or weak because of the low price sensitivity of poorly informed and highly insured patients.

Stephen Shortell and Edward Hughes (1988) performed an exploratory study showing that competition and regulation both lead to poor mortality results. By competition, the authors mean the presence of more than three hospitals within 15 miles. Both CON regulation and hospital rate regulation were associated with higher mortality. If one believes that simply putting hospitals under financial stress would reduce quality and worsen mortality, the finding on CON is problematical. By protecting the hospitals from entry, CON should raise quality, not lower it. The Shortell and Hughes paper contains little theoretical interpretation to explain this finding.

Theories of Hospital Competition

Essentially, there are three competing theories of hospital competition. These are oligopoly and monopolistic competition, redundant resources, and increasing monopoly.

Oligopoly and Monopolistic Competition Theory. The first theory to be considered is the traditional economic theory of oligopoly. Several standard oligopoly theories state that the presence of more competitors leads to more price competition and lower prices (for a constant-quality output). Examples include the theory of George Stigler (1968, 39–66), stressing collusion, and theories stressing oligopolistic interaction without collusion, such as those of Cournot or Bertrand (Carlton and Perloff 1990, 261–76). The standard general theory does not predict whether more competition will raise or lower quality. A more structured variant of the theory proposed by Gregory Pope (1989), however, suggests that nonprice competition will promote quality and administrative efficiency, especially for nonprofit hospitals.

The empirical evidence shows that more competitors lead to more nonprice competition. Some of this nonprice competition is self-defeating from the viewpoint of the industry as a whole (that is, it reduces total profits). Therefore, hospitals have an incentive to collude to suppress nonprice competition. Reducing nonprice competition under the rhetoric of "reducing wasteful duplication" is the main goal of local hospital planning and regulation.

This outcome is not surprising; the complexity of the product makes it difficult for price collusion to be successful. Thus, one would expect that collusion regarding visible technology, equipment, and services would be significantly easier to enforce compared with collusion on the prices of services. Most known collusions focused on easily observable output features such as the number of beds or specific services such as maternity care.

Monopolistic competition. The oligopoly theory applied to hospitals is one of heterogeneous products. In the model of differentiated oligopoly, having a large number of sellers makes it similar to the model of monopolistic competition in which the interactions among rivals disappear from view. In larger cities it makes good sense to apply the model to hospitals (Phelps and Sened 1989). The qualitative predictions of this theory are identical to the oligopoly model. Thus, this model can be considered a variant of the traditional oligopoly model of hospital behavior.

Redundant Resources Theory. The second theory, well described by David Salkever (1978), stresses the physician's influence over patient choices. To attract physicians, hospitals compete through nonprice means like high-tech equipment, more personnel, and more capacity (lower occupancy). More competition among hospitals leads to more intense nonprice competition and raises quality and costs.

Heavily insured consumers are assumed to ignore prices. Thus, hospitals raise prices to maintain profits at some target level as increased nonprice competition raises their costs. This theory implies that more competitors would cause quality to rise but would not change price competition. Therefore, the price of a constant-quality hospital day would not change, nor would profits. Similar results occur when physicians control the hospital, as analyzed by Mark Pauly and Michael Redisch (1973). In their model, increased competition for physicians allows them to use more complementary inputs, such as nursing, which push hospital costs upward. This situation also allows physicians to increase their incomes. This is called the *redundant re-*

sources theory because hospitals compete for physicians by adding resources.

Increasing Monopoly and Search. The third theory is an application of Mark Satterthwaite's increasing monopoly theory (1979) to the hospital market. If overlap in recommendations is necessary for the consumer to have confidence in his information, it follows that information can be worse where there are more alternatives. With more alternatives, the consumer is less likely to receive overlapping recommendations about any providers. If that happens, the presence of more sellers can reduce competition and drive the price of a constant-quality hospital day up and increase profits. Satterthwaite showed that this was possible in a simple computer simulation of a hypothetical market. This model has no predictions for nonprice competition.

A variant of the information-theoretic model comes from Joseph Stiglitz (1987): if search costs are higher for more search, then prices can actually rise with an increase in the number of sellers in the market. The cost of search rises with an increase in the number of firms and thus reduces the consumers' search effort and reduces the elasticity of demand at the level of the individual firm.

Several studies of actual medical shopping behavior and referral networks have shed light on how consumers collect information on medical markets. Alan Booth and Nicholas Babchuk (1972) found patients turning to friends and family for recommendations 73 percent of the time. Thus, they argued that "physicians play a far less important role in the selection of health services than common wisdom and previous research might suggest" (1972, 92). Nancy Howell Lee (1969) studied the sources of information and the chain of search for a physician to perform an abortion. She found that information passed through an average of 2.8 individuals to reach the patient and that the patient had an average of 2.9 physicians to choose from. Wolinsky and Steiber (1982) found considerable support for the importance of social networks and the lay referral system. They concluded that physicians are not as dominant as the literature suggests. The literature "should be expanded to include some measures of both the quantity and information quality of the social networks available to individuals" (1982, 765). Both variants of the information theoretic approach show that adding more hospitals to compete in the same market might reduce competition, rather than increase it.

Issues in Empirical Research

Geographical Market Area. Geographical markets must be defined for studies of local competition. Market definition is a fundamental necessity for antitrust policy, especially toward mergers. The antitrust question is this: Which sellers can constrain the higher prices or lower quality of a hospital or colluding group of hospitals? Such a market includes the sellers from the smallest geographic area who can, in concert, exert market power. Within the market, a hypothetical cartel could profitably raise prices significantly above the competitive level for some period. In its merger guidelines, the U.S. Department of Justice (1992) has suggested using a 5 percent price increase for one or two years. This definition makes sense for most cross-sectional statistical analysis, at least as a conceptual starting point. Actual empirical studies use a variety of market definitions.

Many studies define a market area as either a standard metropolitan statistical area (SMSA) or a county. An exception, Henry Zaretsky (1984), used only California data and used the health facilities planning area as a market area. This mimics small SMSAs (where the SMSA seems a reasonable market area) but breaks up the larger SMSAs into smaller areas. San Francisco and the four surrounding counties, for example, contain eleven health facilities planning areas.

Hal Luft and Susan Maerki (1984–1985) used a purely distance-oriented market definition. Beginning with each hospital's location (actually the location of its post office), Luft and Maerki calculated the number of hospitals within a 15-mile radius of each hospital. They then examined how the presence of more competitors within this radius altered hospital behavior.

This measure overcomes the problem of the large SMSA, although it still has some shortcomings. It ignores the relationship of markets to geographic attributes (mountains, lakes), ease of transport (freeways, mass transit), and employment and shopping patterns. These factors are considered in SMSA definitions, which are designed to reflect local markets. Also, hospitals vary in size and attractiveness, features not accounted for in the Luft and Maerki measure.

These approaches are sometimes justified by an appeal to patient origin studies showing that local market areas are self-contained; that is, there is little export or import of hospital services from the defined local market area. Several studies explicitly define market areas based on patient flow statistics (Morrisey, Sloan, and Valvona 1988; Robinson and Phibbs 1990; Phibbs and Carson 1989; Dranove, Shanley, and Simon 1991). Individual hospital markets for antitrust cases are defined partly by using patient origin studies.

Patient origin statistics are helpful, but they must be used carefully. Taken at face value, they often suggest market areas that are too large compared with the ideal market area of the merger guidelines. Some patients travel long distances from small towns to larger ones to use hospitals of higher quality or hospitals that offer esoteric services unavailable in the small-town hospitals. The direction of this patient flow is hierarchical, moving up the hierarchy of city size and hospital sophistication and generally skipping over nearby towns of equal or smaller size. Some residents of Santa Barbara, for example, go to famous research hospitals in San Francisco or Los Angeles for special services, but there is little flow in the opposite direction.

Patient migration patterns lead some observers, such as Morrisey, Sloan, and Valvona (1988) to suggest that small-town hospitals ought to be included in the market with the sophisticated hospitals in the larger cities. But this would be a mistake. Consumers are not willing to change their decision in response to small price differences among these very different hospitals (Frech 1987; Baker 1988). Gregory Werden (1989) showed formally that the lower-quality distant hospitals do not discipline the prices of the sophisticated hospitals in the central cities. I would argue that the reverse is also true. Dranove, Shanley, and Simon (1991) explicitly modeled this flow up the hierarchy. They found that the competition among distant hospitals was weaker than competition among local ones.

Time Period. The time period of the data is potentially important and interesting because of recent trends toward more procompetitive forms of health insurance (for example, higher consumer copayment, HMOs, and PPOs). Further, profit-seeking hospitals and hospital chains have grown rapidly in recent years. These are widely believed to compete more aggressively. More recent studies of competition would reflect these environmental changes and would be expected to find more price competition.

The Measure of Concentration. There is a long history of research relating the concentration of sellers or buyers to various measures of economic performance, such as price or profits. This requires a measure for concentration.[6] Two types of simple measures are commonly used. The older measure is the concentration ratio, the proportion or percentage of the industry's output that is sold by some number of the largest firms. Traditionally, four-firm and eight-firm concentration ratios have been used, partly because the Bureau of the Census reports them. In hospital markets an eight-firm concentration ratio would not be useful since most urban markets have eight or fewer hospitals. Per-

---

6. See George Stigler (1968, chap. 4) for a discussion of the measurement of concentration.

haps a three-firm concentration ratio would be best for urban hospital markets.

There are several theoretical objections to the concentration ratio. The number of firms used in the definition is arbitrary. Most important, the ratio ignores the distribution of sales among the larger firms and among the smaller ones. These objections gave rise to the Herfindahl index, which takes account of the entire size distribution. It is defined as the sum of squared market shares of the firms in the industry:

$$\text{Herfindahl index} = s_1^2 + s_2^2 + s_3^2 + \ldots + s_n^2 \qquad (3\text{-}1)$$

where s_i is the market share of firm i. Thus, if we measure the market shares as proportions, the Herfindahl index varies from a maximum of one (1.0^2) to a minimum of zero.

The index for a market of three firms of equal size, for example, is 0.3333, or ($0.333^2 + 0.333^2 + 0.333^2$). If two of those firms were to merge, the Herfindahl would become 0.5556 ($0.667^2 + 0.333^2$). The difference is about 0.22. This difference will be called the *benchmark* or *standard merger* in later discussion.[7] Hospital mergers with this effect on the Herfindahl index have been challenged by the antitrust enforcement agencies.[8] The Herfindahl index also can be expressed in percentages, rather than proportions, as the U.S. Department of Justice does. If so, the above values would be 5,556, 3,333, and 2,223.

The Herfindahl index is popular, partly because the Department of Justice has adopted it and partly because it seems somehow more scientific than the simple concentration ratios. Certain oligopoly models can be constructed where the Herfindahl index is the appropriate measure of concentration. But appearances are misleading. One could just as easily construct oligopoly models in which another measure was superior (Carlton and Perloff 1990, 369–70). Most important, empirical research in many national industries over many years has shown that the Herfindahl index is highly correlated with the concentration ratios. In my empirical research, I have found the same to be

---

7. The 1992 merger guidelines of the Department of Justice call for investigations of mergers that raise the Herfindahl index, in terms of percentages, by 100 points or more. In the context of hospital markets, applying this threshold would require an investigation of virtually every hospital merger. In a market with five equally sized hospitals, for example, the Herfindahl would be 2,000 (0.2 by the proportional measure). A merger of two of these would raise it by 800, fully eight times the threshold, to 2,800. Still, at 2,800, this would be a less concentrated hospital market than the U.S. average for SMSAs.

8. Erwin Blackstone and Joseph Fuhr (1989) argue that most mergers challenged by the FTC or the Justice Department were indeed harmful. Thomas Campbell and James Teevans (1991) take the opposite view.

true for cross sections of local hospital markets. Therefore, it usually makes little difference which measure one uses.

Studies of hospital competition have examined the effects of concentration on hospital costs, typically average cost per admission or per day; hospital prices, usually measured by average revenue per inpatient day; the rate of technological diffusion; occupancy rates; and measures of nonprice competition. A few of the more recent analyses have more reasonable measures of hospital prices. Studies analyzing average costs or revenues have necessarily ignored variations in effects on the type of service supplied. Hospitals facing competition may choose, for example, to reduce laboratory prices and simultaneously to raise daily room charges.

Further, appropriate market areas are not independent of the variable studied. Hospitals compete among a tighter circle for more routine procedures and services while competition among open heart surgical facilities undoubtedly crosses state lines in some areas. Consumers are more willing to travel great distances for small improvements in quality or sophistication of services for more serious illnesses (Morrisey, Sloan, and Valvona 1988; Dranove and Shanley 1990; Phibbs and Carson 1989).

Results of Empirical Research

Nonprice Competition. There is much evidence that lower concentration (more competitors) increases nonprice competition, thus quality and cost.[9]

Technological diffusion. Several studies have considered the effects of hospital competition on the choice of new technologies by hospitals. In a comprehensive study of this issue, Louise Russell (1979) considered the effects of concentration, measured by the four-firm concentration ratio. With a sample of 2,772 short-term nonfederal hospitals and using an SMSA market area definition, she analyzed the years in which a hospital opened facilities for major new technologies, such as respiration therapy, diagnostic radioisotopes, electroencephalography, and intensive care. In addition, Russell examined the effects of competition on the number of intensive care hospital beds and whether a hospital had cobalt therapy, open heart surgery, and renal dialysis facilities.

The results were mixed. Market concentration had little of a statistically significant impact. With the year of adoption of a specific technology as a dependent variable, hospitals in markets with a

---

9. For an earlier survey of this literature, see Woolley and Frech (1988–1989).

concentration ratio between 0.50 and 0.79 delayed longest in all four cases, while both more and less concentrated markets seemed to adopt the technology more quickly. Competition had no statistically significant effect on the proportion of beds devoted to intensive care or on the probability of a hospital's offering cobalt therapy or inpatient renal dialysis. Open heart surgery facilities, a prestige technology, seemed significantly more common in more competitive markets, a result consistent with a high degree of nonprice competition for patients or physicians.

John Rappaport (1978), analyzing only urban market areas, found evidence that nuclear medicine technology spread faster in states with less concentrated hospital markets. Anthony Romeo, Judith Wagner, and Robert Lee (1984) found mixed results: lower hospital concentration seemed to reduce the probability of the availability of electronic fetal monitoring and centralized management systems technology, while increasing the availability of volumetric infusion pumps. Robert Lee and Donald Waldman (1985) repeated the analysis of Romeo, Wagner, and Lee with an improved estimator and found considerably different results: only one technology spread more slowly in less concentrated markets, fiberoptic endoscopes. Frank Sloan and others (1986) found diffusion of surgical technology to be less likely in less concentrated markets, which suggests that nonprice competition is not so important.

Harold Luft, Susan Maerki, and Joan Trauner (1986) found that hospitals react in competitive or complementary fashions, depending on the service. They found that hospitals are more likely to have mammography, twenty-four-hour emergency care, and cardiac catheterization if their competitors have them but are less likely to offer cobalt therapy or heart surgery.

The effect of more nearby competitors in reducing the chance of a hospital's using the last two technologies makes sense. Hospitals probably chose a complementary strategy for cobalt therapy because only a few radiation therapy specialists use cobalt equipment. Such a facility would not attract many new physicians. Cobalt therapy equipment may be prohibitively expensive unless the hospital can expect most of the business in an area. Also, cobalt treatment is typically performed on an outpatient basis so that the equipment would not increase hospital inpatient admissions by much.

The complementary strategy for open heart surgery units is probably due to the perception that outcomes are better in a high-volume setting. Both hospitals and local health care planning agencies favor limiting the number of open heart units in each market area. Only about 10 percent of the nation's hospitals did heart surgery in 1972, and these were usually regionally dispersed.

James Robinson, Deborah Garnick, and Stephen McPhee (1987) investigated the spread of heart units. They analyzed the influence of competition and regulation on the availability of percutaneous transluminal coronary angioplasty and coronary-artery bypass surgery in 1983. If we control for case mix, teaching role, and population, hospitals with more than twenty competitors (clearly, all in large cities) were 155 percent more likely to offer coronary angioplasty and 147 percent more likely to offer bypass surgery than those with no competitors. Both findings were statistically significant. The probability of either being the result of chance was less than one in ten thousand. They concluded that competition encouraged and regulation discouraged the proliferation of these cardiac services. In sum, lower concentration (more competitors) seems to lead hospitals to introduce most new technologies sooner.

Costs and services. Many studies have examined the effect of more competitors on services available to hospital consumers. Paul Joskow (1982), using data from 1977, studied the effects of competition on reservation margins for hospital beds (the ability to be sure that a bed will be available). He argued that hospitals with more competitors would be more concerned with guaranteeing immediate patient access to hospital beds. Joskow's empirical results showed that concentration had a statistically and economically significant effect on reducing the reserve margin of hospitals.

Joskow used estimates from the literature on the costs of an empty bed to argue that this higher capacity is expensive and probably wasteful. But Bernard Friedman and Mark Pauly (1981) have shown that the long-run cost of a hospital bed expected to be empty is low, about 8 percent of the cost of a full bed. The previous studies Joskow relied on had erred because they were unable to isolate long-run costs.

If a hospital expects a bed to be empty, it chooses a low level of inputs (for example, nursing, administrative, housekeeping staff) appropriately, so costs are low. Conversely, if a hospital expects that a particular bed will be filled, it chooses a higher level of inputs to care for the patient so costs will be higher. On short notice, a hospital cannot adjust its inputs fully. In the extreme, if there were no notice at all, costs of an unexpectedly empty bed would be close to 100 percent of those of an occupied bed. Earlier empirical work, simply relating occupancy rate to accounting costs, captures some mixture of expectedly and unexpectedly empty beds. Philip Hersch (1982, 1984) found that lower concentration led to more hospital care, as measured by expenditures, registered nurses (RNs), and licensed practical nurses (LPNs) per day of care. He used 1972 data. He also found that increased competition led to longer average durations of patient stay. Certificate-of-need legislation was found to preserve market structure and to reduce competition. Unfortunately, he was unable to examine the effects of competition on prices.

George Wilson and Joseph Jadlow (1982) related costs of nuclear medicine departments to ownership and to hospital concentration within local markets. They found costs higher in more competitive local markets. These results should be viewed as suggestive only, because of the empirical model used.

Wilson and Jadlow measured hospital concentration by a three-way interaction of hospital density, referral radius (of the individual hospital), and population density. In addition, they used the frontier production function approach, which amounts to assuming that the lower-cost hospitals are efficient.[10] They also found that profit-seeking hospitals had lower costs than private nonprofit or governmental hospitals.

A study by James Robinson and Harold Luft (1985) used 1972 data to examine the effect of more competitors on patient volume, length of stay, and cost (as measured by cost per patient and cost per patient day). With the pure distance market definition (the number of hospitals within 15 miles), they analyzed 5,013 general hospitals nationwide and corrected for case mix and quality variation by using American Hospital Association service variables.

To allow for detailed case mix corrections based on diagnostic data, they examined a smaller sample of 1,084 hospitals. Controlling for this better measure of case mix changed little in the coefficients on the numbers of competitors: either the AHA survey variables are reasonable proxies for case mix and quality or variation in case mix and quality is not empirically important. This finding increases confidence in the rest of the literature.

Robinson and Luft found evidence that the presence of more competitors increased hospital admissions and total per capita hospital costs. This effect of market structure on per capita costs by area has not been studied much; further work would be valuable.

---

10. In statistical terms, the frontier production method assumes that the error term is asymmetrical because all errors in management lead to costs that are higher than those of the efficient firms. Since there are other important sources of error, such as case mix and quality variation, this assumption is probably inappropriate. Further, the actual distribution of hospital costs and the residuals from fitting hospital cost functions do not show the asymmetry suggested by the production frontier approach.

Hospitals with one neighbor reported costs 6 percent higher than hospitals with no neighbors; those with two to four neighbors reported costs 9 percent higher; those with five to ten neighbors reported costs 16–17 percent higher; and those with more than ten neighbors reported costs 20–21 percent higher. Hospitals with greater average lengths of stay reported higher costs per admission but lower costs per patient day, as expected.[11] Higher levels of admissions, which are associated with higher occupancy rates, also led to lower daily costs, as expected. The study included some controls on demand variables but excluded demographic variables.

At least in this older data, the presence of more competitors is associated with higher costs. This factor supports the idea of nonprice competition for physicians or patients. But markets with higher physician-to-population ratios reported significantly higher costs per admission and per inpatient day. This is evidence against the view that when physicians are scarce, competition for their favor drives up costs. This also serves as evidence against the idea that physicians act as substitutes for inpatient care.

Hospitals in areas with more inpatient days per capita also have lower costs, a result consistent with the effect of price on the selection of patients to hospitalize. The effect was fairly strong, with an elasticity of about -0.084, indicating that a 10 percent increase in use reduces costs per day by nearly 1 percent. This finding is also consistent with simply moving down the demand curve so that areas with lower hospital prices have greater utilization.

This study is unusual in finding that profit-seeking hospitals have lower costs (by 7.6 percent) than nonprofit ones, when number of competitors, case mix, and hospital days per population are controlled for (Robinson and Luft 1985, 348, 349). The finding is statistically significant at the 1 percent level. Perhaps other studies have erred by not holding those variables constant.

Charity care. One would expect that more competition among hospitals would reduce the potential monopoly rents available to cross-subsidize activities favored by the hospital decision makers. Thus, some have feared a reduction in charity care provided to the poor as competition increases. In a study relating hospital concentration to the supply of charity care by nonprofit hospitals, Richard Frank and David Salkever (1991) found just the opposite. They hypothesized that one

---

11. Because the first days of care are typically the most intensive and costly, average cost per day would be expected to decline with increased average length of stay.

element of nonprice competition among hospitals is charity care, so that more competing hospitals in a market area lead to more charity care. This fascinating finding deserves to be tested further. Perhaps when and if competition becomes strong enough, the reduction in available monopoly rents will dominate, and the result will be reversed.

Price Competition. There are fewer studies of hospital pricing and price competition because price data are harder to obtain. Still, the available studies tell a consistent story. Using 1982 data, a study done for a hospital antitrust case by Henry Zaretsky (1984) presents some interesting results. Examining California markets and correcting concentration measures to account for multihospital ownership and management, he found a weak negative effect of concentration on net revenue per patient day.

By confining his study to California, Zaretsky was able to use the health facilities planning area as a market area. This is a unique feature of his research. Using a Herfindahl index of market concentration, he found that an increase in the index of 0.22 (the equivalent of the two hospitals merging in a market initially characterized by three equal-sized hospitals) would lead to a net revenue reduction of about 4.5 percent. Zaretsky also found the occupancy rate to have a strong positive effect on net revenue, even though high occupancy rates are known to reduce average costs. This finding is consistent with research in many industries. High occupancy or capacity utilization rates weaken the incentive to compete on price. If firms are close to their capacity limits, a price cut cannot be rewarded by a large increase in sales. While Zaretsky's study is informative, there are some problems with it: it did not adjust for most market and hospital characteristics.

Zaretsky's variable for price is what hospitals call *net revenue,* total charges minus discounts to some payers and bad debts. If it were not for the bad debts, it would measure the price consumers get with the average discount. Many consumers receive no discount. There is no perfect measure of price.

Zaretsky treated hospitals under common ownership or management in the same market as a single hospital in calculating the concentration index. While the adjustment for common ownership is correct, it is problematic to view all hospitals using the same hospital management firm as if they were one. Such hospitals may not coordinate pricing, quality, or amenity decisions in monopolistic ways. Nonprofit hospitals owned by religious bodies may be especially unlikely to coordinate decision making with profit-seeking hospital management companies that own competitors. A close examination of the role of the hospitals' boards of directors and medical staffs and the management contracts would be necessary to decide whether to treat the managed firms as if they were combined.

Dean Farley (1985) studied the effect of the number of competitors on revenue per patient day and other financial variables. Using a sample of 400 short-term, general, nonfederal hospitals in the United States from 1970 to 1977, Farley found that hospitals in markets with more competitors produce significantly more expensive medical care than those in single-hospital markets. Hospitals in counties with at least four competitors had 27.81 percent higher operating expenses and earned 17.61 percent greater gross revenues (per adjusted admission) than hospitals with a monopoly in their county.

The presence of more competitors raises costs far more than price and implies lower hospital margins and more price competition. Hospitals in markets with more competitors employed more capital and labor, offered more services and performed more procedures, had longer lengths of stay, and maintained lower occupancy rates. Hospital services in less concentrated areas were clearly more service-intensive and more sophisticated, as measured by the availability of specialized services. To the extent that quality is measured or proxied by sophistication of services, higher quality characterizes the hospitals in more competitive markets. Unfortunately, Farley failed to account for various influences on health care outcomes including insurance levels and corrects for demographic characteristics only by a variable for each of sixty-four regions.

Farley's price measure, gross revenue per admission, is the opposite of Zaretsky's. Though valid and useful, it is also imperfect; it measures the price paid by those who cannot obtain discounts. While more than half the population in 1977 paid list price, not everyone did.

Monica Noether's studies (1987, 1988) also cover price competition. She examined both price and nonprice competition in a study of about 2,800 hospitals located in SMSAs in 1977 and 1978. Noether obtained a reasonable price measure, average hospital charges per admission, for eleven disease categories. This is a gross measure, before discounts are subtracted. The data came from Health Care Financing Administration files of average charges and are derived from a 20 percent sample of Medicare hospital inpatient bills. While the price data intrinsically control for case mix, one would like to hold quality constant as well.

Lower concentration, as measured by the Herfindahl index, had a positive effect on ten of the eleven prices but was statistically insignificant in all equations at the 95 percent level. The small estimated coefficients show that concentration had little impact on hospital prices.

Averaging over all eleven diagnoses, Noether (1987, 69) found that an increase in the Herfindahl index of 0.22 reduced the price by only 0.77 percent when estimated at the SMSA level and by 1.17 percent when estimated at the level of the individual hospital.

Conversely, hospital expenses per admission did significantly decrease in more concentrated markets, falling by 5.94 or 3.74 percent for the same 0.22 increase in the Herfindahl index. Noether stated that her result "suggests that hospital margins rise and expenses fall with increases in hospital industry concentration (reduced competition), where expenses are interpreted as reflecting quality. It therefore appears that normal competitive forces affect the hospital industry" (1987, 81). She also found that certificate-of-need laws have led to higher prices and expenses. States with such laws for ten years or longer had 8.3 percent higher prices and 7.7 percent higher expenses. In addition, profit-seeking hospitals charged higher prices (although their expenses were not significantly different from nonprofit hospitals). She maintained that their presence did not seem to increase price competition.

This last conclusion is suspect because of selection bias. Empirical research by Ross Mullner and Jack Hadley (1984) shows that profit-seeking hospitals select higher-priced markets to enter. Selection alone would cause the proportion of profit-seeking hospitals to be correlated with higher prices. If so, a positive correlation between profit-seeking hospitals and prices is possible, even if they did encourage price competition.

Noether found that HMO membership and growth did not have a statistically significant effect on hospital prices or costs. She noted that this is expected to change in more recent years. She also found that the presence of more physicians, either per bed or per capita in the market, raises prices and costs. This finding is consistent with the other literature.

Another study of hospital competition, prices, and costs was done by J. Michael Woolley and H. E. Frech (Woolley 1987; Woolley and Frech 1992). This analysis focused on consumer information. It used actual prices for hospital daily charges and several ancillary services. In common with many studies, this one used the SMSA as the market definition. Data were aggregated to the SMSA level.

The year 1970 was picked as the year least likely to offer evidence of price competition. Hospital insurance was near its peak of completeness in 1970; also, 1970 predated the explosive growth of HMOs, PPOs, and other kinds of managed care.

Using a fairly complete econometric model like Noether's, Frech and Woolley confirmed her results. The existence of fewer competitors (more concentration) reduced hospital daily room and board prices slightly, raised prices for ancillary services, but reduced costs, and presumably quality, by much more. In the analysis most comparable to Noether's, a 0.22 increase in the Herfindahl index was found to reduce costs by 2.9 percent (statistically significant at the 95 percent level), while it had a smaller, 1.5 percent (statistically significant at only the 70 percent level) effect in reducing daily room and board charges.

The effect on the prices of six ancillary (laboratory) services was decidedly different. Here, the traditional oligopoly theory was borne out. Higher concentration was associated with higher prices. On average, a 0.22 increase in the Herfindahl index raised these prices by 2.5 percent. These findings were reasonably strong, with statistical significance varying from the 99 percent level to the 62 percent level. The more accurately estimated effects were the largest.

Frech and Woolley included variables to capture the level of consumer information (the proportion of female-headed households, the proportion of households with a telephone, and the proportion of households that recently moved). Following expectations these information variables were more important in the price equations than the cost equations. As a block, they were statistically significant at the 84 percent level in the daily charges regression and much more important in the ancillary fee equations, exceeding the 99 percent level in four of the six price equations. The signs, as expected, were positive for the female-headed households and negative for possession of a telephone. The proportion who moved consistently showed a negative effect on price, the opposite of what was expected.

This result may be caused by selection. Moving is a costly investment in a better future. The economics literature often treats migration as an investment in human capital. Thus, consumers who have recently moved are younger and better educated than those who have not. The movers may also be more productive in searching for health care providers, despite the disadvantage of a recent move. In any event, more research on the relationship between consumer information and the proportion of consumers who have recently moved would be useful. The evidence thus suggests that increasing concentration reduces costs and quality levels by reducing nonprice competition but has little net effect on prices when both daily room and ancillary service charges are considered.

Frech and Woolley went on to estimate the effects of concentration on nonprice competition or quality directly, as measured by an index of available services. They found strong effects. Nonprice competition is reduced as concentration increases. This suggests that the price of a constant-quality hospital day may be higher in more concentrated markets, though the price of the average hospital day may be lower. The occupancy rate was negatively related to both average costs and price (Woolley 1987, 130–32). The effect on costs is about three times the effect on price. The small negative effect on price was the opposite of what Zaretsky found.

Higher occupancy rates have two effects. First, they discourage competition, since a hospital with high occupancy can increase its sales only a limited amount by dropping its price. Second, higher occupancy rates reduce average costs, while raising marginal costs. Woolley's finding that higher occupancy rates are correlated with lower prices suggests an element of average cost pricing. This pricing requires the persistence of some unexploited market power, at least for some hospitals. The finding that only about one-third of the saving in average costs is passed on to consumers suggests that hospital pricing cannot be explained as average cost plus a markup.

The pattern in the studies using older data is clear. Greater hospital concentration (fewer competitors) reduces nonprice competition. Costs and measures of quality (services) decline. Simultaneously, higher hospital concentration reduces price competition. The cost savings from reduced nonprice competition are partly but not fully passed on to consumers. This suggests that a hospital merger within a market area ought to decrease both types of hospital competition and to increase hospital profits.

Financial Market Evidence. There are problems in the accounting data used in the above studies of costs. Perhaps the most serious is the treatment of capital costs. Depreciation charges are inherently arbitrary. The correct opportunity cost for owners' equity is not clear. Fortunately, there is another method to test whether mergers increase the monopoly power of the remaining hospitals. Woolley (1989, 1991) has used this approach. He examined the effects of twenty-three events, seventeen promerger and six antimerger, from 1969 through 1985, on the stock prices of profit-seeking hospital corporations.

Stock price data have many advantages over accounting data. They are free of the complex biases and errors of accounting data. Further, they are forward looking. Changes in stock prices reflect the judgment of expert investors about the long-run effects of an event. A merger, for example, may be expected to lead to less competition as investment decisions are made but with little or no immediate changes. If so, the stock price would rise immediately to reflect higher expected profits, while accounting data would not reflect the reduced competition for some time. There are many possible reasons for firms to merge, and most of them (for example, greater efficiency, poor management)

43

would increase the value of the merging firms. Thus, one cannot infer anything from the changes in the stock prices of the merging firms.

Changes in the stock prices of the competitors of the merged firms can differentiate mergers for efficiency from mergers for monopoly. The merged firms must raise prices or reduce quality and amenities to exercise their enhanced market power. This action raises the profits of the competing hospitals. To examine this, Woolley constructed portfolios of all publicly traded hospital corporations except those that are merging. Eliminating marketwide stock price variations enhances the statistical power of the technique. Woolley used the standard capital asset model of modern finance theory to control for the effects of the market as a whole.

He found that mergers raised the profitability of the nonmerging hospital firms. In twelve of the seventeen promerger events, the stock of competing hospital firms rose. In five of the six antimerger events, the stock of the nonmerging hospitals fell. These results are statistically significant at levels ranging from 90 to 98 percent. Woolley also found that the mergers raised stock prices more when the merging firms had more hospitals in the same geographical markets. Thus, financial data show that hospital mergers typically reduce price and nonprice competition.

Insurance Innovations, PPOs, and HMOs. The increasing popularity of HMOs and PPOs over the past decade should have a dramatic effect on hospital competition. Lawrence Goldberg and Warren Greenberg (1977b) pointed out the necessity of taking HMOs and their effects on competition into account. They showed that HMOs have a strong negative effect on Blue Cross hospital utilization rates and increase hospital service competition. Frech (1988b) described how PPOs can improve consumer information and thus stimulate competition.

The effect of HMOs on hospital competition in Minneapolis-St. Paul has been studied. Using data from the late 1970s and early 1980s, Harold Luft and others (1986) found that HMOs failed to reduce hospital use and, because of employee self-selection, apparently raised employer costs (at least in selected instances). This last conclusion is tentative because of data limitations.

Allan Johnson and David Aquilina (1986) found that, through 1981, HMO growth had not significantly affected total hospital costs, revenues, or profits. They argued that competition would not be promoted if "the major buyers of hospital care, HMOs included, do not reward cost-containing behavior by directing patients to cost-effective hospitals instead of shopping for discounts which merely shift higher prices to other payers" (672).

This is a strange argument. Why should buyers care about the costs of sellers? The price and quality are all they care about. The high-cost sellers must eventually reduce costs to meet the market price. The finding that discounting hospitals do not have lower costs is surprising, but it has nothing to do with the advantages or disadvantages of competition. Further, the discounting hospitals may be of higher quality so that they have a lower cost per constant-quality hospital day than the other hospitals.

Roger Feldman, Bryan Dowd, Don McCann, and Allan Johnson (1986) found that hospitals granting larger HMO discounts did not have lower costs per admission. They suggested that these discounts do not force hospitals to act more efficiently. Hospitals with disproportionately large payments from HMOs, Medicare, and Medicaid had the same costs per admission as other hospitals, casting doubt on whether the discounts were based on cost savings. Finally, HMO market share had no significant adverse effect on hospital profits.

In contrast, James Robinson (1991) found that hospital cost inflation within California was lower in market areas with higher HMO market shares. He also found the ability of all insurers to contract selectively with hospitals was important in reducing costs.

Taken together, these results indicate that HMOs do reduce hospital cost increases but the effects are not immediate and higher market shares (such as those found in California) are helpful. More research on this topic would be worthwhile.

Insurance reform and more price competition. As predicted, insurance reforms in recent years have made price competition more important (Frech and Ginsburg 1978a; Dranove, Satterthwaite, and Sindelar 1986). Recent analyses—Glenn Melnick and Jack Zwanziger (1989), Zwanziger and Melnick (1988), James Robinson and Harold Luft (1988), and Dranove, Shanley, and White (1991)—show that innovations in health insurance have favored competition. HMOs, PPOs, higher hospital copayments, and competitive bidding by Medicaid have changed the nature of competition, in emphasizing price more than in the past. This change has reduced the growth of cost and price more in less concentrated local markets.

Melnick and Zwanziger used California data to study the impact of lower hospital concentration on the rate of increase of hospital costs from 1980 to 1982, before legislation allowed insurers and required MediCal (California's Medicaid) to contract selectively with hospitals on price. They compared this with the rate of increase from 1982 to 1986. The authors used a novel geographical market definition. They defined each individual hospital's market area as the set of ZIP Code areas from which it drew at least 3 percent of its inpatients. Next, they calculated the Herfindahl indexes for these areas. Finally, they defined the top quartile as low-competition markets and the bottom quartile as high-competition markets.

They found that hospital inflation in the state was lower in the later period. Most important, they found that, during the later period, cost inflation was lower, by 3.53 percent, in the less concentrated (more competitive) local markets. They attributed the difference to MediCal selective contracting, but there were other concurrent developments in private health insurance. HMOs and especially PPOs experienced explosive growth. Simultaneously, consumer copayments for hospital care rose rapidly. As these developments continue, even more hospital competition is likely to focus on price and cost.

Robinson and Luft (1988) performed a similar analysis, although they used a pure-distance market definition and examined hospitals nationally as well as within California. They found that hospitals with more competitors had higher costs in both 1982 and 1986 but that the difference narrowed over time in all states, as a reflection of more pro-competitive hospital insurance. Interestingly, they found a bigger change in California. By 1986 hospitals with more competitors no longer had higher costs. They attributed this to California's policies allowing selective contracting by hospital insurers. Lower costs in more competitive areas are partly due to a tendency for hospitals to specialize more (Farley and Hogan 1990; Dranove and White 1990).

To date, only one study has examined the effect of the more price-competitive environment in California on pricing rather than on costs. Dranove, Shanley, and White (1991) found that price inflation was greater in more concentrated markets within California from 1983 to 1988, after the procompetitive legal and market changes.

Physician and Hospital Interaction. Research on physician-hospital interaction is far from complete. In an early demand study, Joseph Newhouse and Charles Phelps (1976) found physician and hospital care to be gross complements. Higher physician prices discouraged hospitalization, based on nonexperimental econometric results. The RAND Corporation experiment (Newhouse et al. 1981; Manning et al. 1987) revealed that a higher deductible for ambulatory care alone reduced hospital use.

Jeffrey McCombs (1984) disagreed; he stressed the correlation of higher physician and population ratios with lower hospital use in cross-sectional nonexperimental studies. But physician and population ratios are endogenous. Thus, I find the experimental results more convincing.

William Custer (1986) examined the physician and hospital relationship from the physician's viewpoint. Hospitals compete for physicians through increases in hospital attributes and decreasing costs of affiliation with the hospital. The affiliation costs consist mostly of physician time donated to the hospital to help administer it. The physician and the hospital compete for the patient both through hospital and physician attributes and through hospital and physician prices. This three-agent model allows the physician's motives to differ from both the hospital's and the patient's.

Using data from 1977, Custer estimated a hedonic price function for physician services. The results show that hospital characteristics have a significant effect on physician prices. Physicians affiliated with hospitals offering more services charge more. Further, hospital competition reduces physician prices. Finally, physician density is negatively related to physician prices, suggesting that an increased supply of physicians lowers physician prices. These results point out the importance of considering the physician's role in hospital competition.

Scale Economies. Most empirical research takes the size distribution of sellers as given or exogenous. One might ask how the size distribution arose. In an ordinary market of profit-seeking firms, the economies or diseconomies of scale help determine the number and sizes of competitors. The difficulties of raising capital for nonprofit hospitals and possible physician influence complicate this relationship. Still, scale economies in the hospital market are worth investigating on a purely scientific basis.

Although information on hospital scale economies is vital for everyday antitrust and especially merger decisions, the statistical literature relating size to production or costs is in disarray.[12] The earlier studies generally reported increasing returns to scale (Pauly 1978a; Evans 1971; Carr and Feldstein 1967; Cohen 1967; Lave and Lave 1970).[13] Studies concentrating on medium and large hospitals found approximately constant returns to scale (Lave, Lave, and Silberman 1972). Carson Bays (1980) and Martin Feldstein (1968) found constant returns to scale when the physician input was included in the analysis. Some newer studies still found increasing returns (Feldman, Dowd, McCann, and Johnson 1986; Vitaliano 1987; Wilson and Jadlow 1982).

---

12. For a survey of the cost and production function studies of hospital costs see Cowing, Holtman, and Powers (1983).

13. The terminology of scale economies can be confusing. Scale economies imply increasing returns to scale. That is, if a firm were to double all inputs, its output would more than double.

But most of the more sophisticated, newer studies found decreasing returns to scale (Jenkins 1980; Friedman and Pauly 1981; Becker and Sloan 1985; Robinson 1985; Robinson and Phibbs 1990). Conversely, industry participants and observers believe that there are scale economies. Even the Antitrust Division of the U.S. Department of Justice shares this belief. When he was assistant attorney general for antitrust, Charles Rule said that the most efficient hospitals ranged in size from 300 to 600 beds (1988, 15). Also, bond-rating companies refuse to rate the bonds of hospitals with fewer than 100 beds.

Another approach to the issue of scale economies can shed light on these findings and reconcile the disparate results: the survivor analysis, originated by George Stigler (1958). In this analysis, one examines changes in the size distribution of firms in an industry. The smallest size that is still growing is considered the minimum efficient scale at which firms are large enough to exploit all scale economies.[14] For medical services, this technique has an advantage over the statistical approaches. It includes all factors that affect the efficiency of the firms, including variations in quality and consumers' costs that cannot be included in accounting data.

This approach has been applied to the hospital industry by Bays (1986), Frech (1988), Frech and Mobley (1995), and Mobley and Frech (1994). Using national data from 1971 to 1977, Bays found that hospitals with fewer than 100 beds were losing market share; thus there were scale economies at sizes below 100 beds. Using data from 1970 to 1985, Frech reached the same result both for the entire United States and for Oregon. Using data from 1980 to 1986, Frech and Mobley had similar results; that is, scale economies existed from about 100 to 300 beds. They also pursued a multivariate econometric version of the survivor analysis, following Theodore Keeler's (1989) approach. This technique allows other variables reflecting hospital and market characteristics to be held constant. The results for scale economies are essentially unchanged. The survivor analyses agree with the industry experts in finding scale economies.

How then can the sophisticated econometrics of cost and production data go wrong? The answer turns on careful consideration of subtle quality and selection differences among hospitals. Let us take

---

14. The standard approach views the size distribution of the firms as approaching an optimal one from some historically given size distribution. Alternatively, if one views the actual size distribution as relatively close to optimal, one can simply take a statistic such as the average size firm as the minimum efficient scale. This approach is often taken in studies using different industries as observations.

up the quality issue first. As viewed by consumers and physicians, larger hospitals provide a higher quality service. Consumers value the larger menu of available services at larger hospitals (Feldman and Dowd 1986; Frech and Woolley 1992; Luft et al. 1990). Further, consumers favor hospitals with better outcomes, and better outcomes are associated with higher surgical volumes (Luft, Garnick, Mark, and McPhee, 1990, 108). Larger hospitals can more easily attain higher volumes.

Patient selection also works to give the appearance, in cost and output statistics, that larger hospitals are less efficient. Larger hospitals, with their more sophisticated offerings, attract the sicker patients, who are more costly to care for. A cost study by James Robinson (1985) gives some insight into this. He discovered that including variables for case mix in his hospital analysis reduced the apparent cost disadvantage of the larger hospitals.

Larger hospitals have higher accounting costs, but not because of inefficient large size. Rather, providing higher quality care to sicker patients causes the costs to rise. When allowing for quality, larger hospitals are more efficient, not less efficient. There are scale economies. The survivorship literature suggests that the scale economies are more important than one would have thought and that they continue up to a size of about 100 to 300 beds.

Directions for Future Research

With new regulation, innovation, and insurance structures, the hospital industry is constantly evolving. Insurance is becoming more procompetitive by increasing consumer copayments and by increased use of PPOs and HMOs. More price-conscious consumers will change the relationship between competition and hospital prices, reducing the importance of nonprice competition and increasing the importance of price competition. Since the basic structure of incentives and consumer information is changing so much, there is always a role for newer, more extensive studies of the industry. As Melnick and Zwanziger (1989) and Robinson and Luft (1988) show, this is already happening.

Appendix 3-A: Hospital Pricing and the Price Elasticity of Demand

To calculate a conservative estimate of the price increase necessary to maximize profits, given the assumption of perfect monopoly, consider the price necessary to get to the boundary of the elastic region. Assuming linear demand and an elasticity of -0.2, we have the following two relations:

$$\eta = \frac{dq}{dp}\frac{p^\circ}{q^\circ} = -b\frac{p^\circ}{q^\circ} = -0.2 \qquad \text{(3A-1)}$$

and

$$q = a - bp \qquad \text{(3A-2)}$$

where

η = price elasticity of demand for hospital care facing the individual hospital and the hospital industry as a whole

p = price of hospital care

q = quantity of hospital care

p° = currently observed price

q° = currently observed quantity

a, b = parameters of the demand function

Given the assumed elasticity of -0.2 and setting $p^\circ = \$1$, $q^\circ = 1.0$ to normalize requires that $b = 0.2$ and $a = b + 1 = 1.2$. Therefore, at a price at the boundary of the elastic region

$$-b\frac{p^1}{q^1} = -1.0. \qquad \text{(3A-3)}$$

Substituting gives

$$\frac{-0.2 \times p^1}{1.2 - 0.2p^1} = -1.0 \qquad \text{(3A-4)}$$

or

$$p^1 = \$3.0,$$

which is three times the currently observed price.

Profit maximizing occurs at a price higher still, since hospital care is hardly costless to produce. In fact, if we assume that the costs were equal to $\$1.00$ per unit, the profit-maximizing price, where marginal revenue is equal to marginal cost, would be $\$3.50$, or 250 percent higher than the observed price.

4
Competition among Physicians

Competition among physicians is not perfect. This imperfection is partly due to such unavoidable factors as the complex nature of the services and costly consumer information. The flawed competition also results partly from the actions of groups of physicians, often supported by state regulation. Federal and state policies have, perhaps inadvertently, encouraged more complete health insurance, which also harms competition.

History of Licensure

Medicine is an old profession, but it did not always command the high status and income it does now in the United States and western Europe. In the Roman Empire, physicians were typically slaves, freedmen, and foreigners because the physician's status and income were too low to attract the Romans themselves (Starr 1982, 6). In the former Soviet Union, the average physician income was below that of the average blue-collar worker. (Interestingly, the percentage of female physicians is far higher in the former Soviet Union than in the United States.)

In the United States, the income and status of physicians were low until the early twentieth century. In 1850, the average income of a Massachusetts physician was estimated at $600 per year. In 1860, the U.S. average nonfarm annual income (including working children and women) was estimated at $363 (Starr 1982, 84). In those days, skilled manual laborers and craftsmen earned more than the average physician.

Contrast those figures with modern statistics. In 1991, mean physician incomes were $170,600, while average annual compensation was $32,649 (U.S. Bureau of the Census 1994, 123, 427). While the gap has been narrowing for the past few years, the long-term growth in the income difference is explained by science, politics, and economics.

In eighteenth-century America, most physicians lacked formal training. Anyone could call himself a doctor and could practice medicine. Many pursued medicine part time. The minority of American physicians with some training organized state and local medical societies and tried to restrict entry into the profession by colonial or state licensure as early as 1760.

These early medical societies argued that licensure was necessary to protect the consumer from fraudulent or incompetent doctors. In some colonies or states they succeeded, but their victories were primarily symbolic. In the eighteenth century, licensing was usually permissive—unlicensed practitioners were also allowed to practice medicine. Today we would call this certification, rather than licensure. A few states prohibited unlicensed physicians from using the courts to collect bad debts (Starr 1982, 35). In practice, this was of little importance. The Canadian Maritime Provinces followed the U.S. example, but the other provinces had stricter licensure throughout the period (Hamowy 1984, 34, 35).

Competing Theories of Disease and Cure. In the eighteenth and nineteenth centuries, physicians held many wildly different theories of disease and medicine. The elite orthodox physicians sought to gain a monopoly for what they considered scientific medicine.

In fact, orthodox medicine was not only unscientific but unhealthy. Benjamin Rush, a revolutionary leader and physician, was typical of orthodox medicine. He taught that there was only one disease in the world, morbid excitement induced by capillary tension. It had one remedy—depleting the body by bleeding and emptying the stomach and bowels by laxatives. Patients were to be bled until they passed out (Starr 1982, 43). Powerful poisons, such as mercury and other minerals, were also part of the standard treatment that was to dominate standard medicine for a hundred years. Orthodox physicians believed that eyeglasses were useless and even harmful well into the nineteenth century (Maurizi, Moore, and Shepard 1981, 354–55). Such was the scientific practice that those physicians sought to protect from competition by licensure.

Alternatives to orthodoxy came into flower in the early nineteenth century. One important example was Samuel Thompson, who, like Rush, taught that there was only one disease, cold, and one cure, heat. Heat was to be produced either directly or by clearing the stomach of obstructions by laxatives so that the digestion of food would cause heat to be released. Bleeding was not part of the regime. Thompsonism was most popular in low-income rural areas.

Homeopathy, in contrast, was most successful among the better-educated and higher-income consumers. It held that diseases could be cured by drugs that caused the same symptoms as the disease, hence the name. Further, the effects of drugs would be heightened by giving them in minute doses. To decide which drugs to use, the doctor had to pay close and sympathetic attention to the patient. In effect, homeopathic treatment was based on the placebo effect. At least it was not harmful, which is more than one can say for orthodox medicine (Starr 1982, 51–54, 96–97). The homeopaths dubbed the orthodox doctors *allopaths* (cure by opposites), a term that stuck and is still in use today.

The Jacksonian Democrats and the Decline of Licensure. Early licensing was repealed under the principled attack of the Jacksonian Democrats in the mid-1800s. They favored open competitive markets and opposed artificial licensed monopolies, including the licensed professions. By 1860, most states had dropped licensure for physicians and lawyers. Illinois is especially amusing because it established physician licensure in 1817 only to repeal it nine years later (Starr 1982, 58). At that time, most medical societies tried to fix prices by promulgating fee schedules, as discussed below.

The American Medical Association and the Revival of Licensure. In this free-entry environment, doctors founded the American Medical Association (AMA) in 1847. It immediately adopted the proposal of Nathan Smith Davies, which called for mandatory state licensure of physicians, with boards dominated by representatives of state medical societies. Graduation from a medical school approved by the medical society would be a prerequisite for licensure. The AMA gradually prevailed. Between 1880 and 1900, every state had adopted licensure dominated by state medical societies (Berlant 1981, 11–14). The Jacksonian Democratic opposition to licensure had evaporated.

But licensure had not restricted entry into the medical profession. Licensure simply channeled entry through the medical schools. From 1880 to 1890, the number of medical students grew from 11,826 to 25,171. The AMA failed to control the entry and expansion of medical schools, largely because the AMA itself was small and weak. The political power rested with the state medical societies. Thus, in 1901 the AMA reorganized as a confederation of state medical societies. This result was dramatic. From 1900 to 1910, membership rose from 8,000 to 70,000 physicians (Starr 1982, 110, 112).

At the same time, membership in the state medical society was becoming more important for physicians. The societies controlled expert witnesses for medical malpractice cases since the standard of due care that the courts used, until recently, was local practice. Also, hospitals were increasingly requiring membership for hospital privileges. Simultaneously, the middle and upper classes began using hospitals.

The Flexner Report and Modern Licensure. After 1910, the medical profession gained control of the medical schools, raised standards, and reduced the number of schools and the number of students. The standard view (Kessel 1958; Rayack 1967) has credited this to a 1910 report on medical schools, *Medical Education in the U.S. and Canada,* written by Abraham Flexner, supported by the Carnegie Foundation for the Advancement of Teaching. Flexner recommended raising standards for medical schools and students and reducing the number of both schools and students. Indeed, the number of medical schools fell from 131 to 76 between 1910 and the final implementation of the report in 1930 (French 1974, 124).[1]

Paul Starr disputes the traditional emphasis on Flexner's role; he notes that the state licensing boards had already begun to raise standards and had eliminated some medical schools before the 1910 report. Whatever their source, the restrictions effectively reduced the supply of physicians from 173 per 100,000 population in 1900 to 125 per 100,000 in 1930 (Starr 1982, 118–23, 126).

Licensure and Discrimination. Because of the elimination of many medical schools and the scaling back of the rest, the competitive position of the remaining schools changed greatly. Instead of actively competing for all the students they could get, the schools started turning away large numbers of applicants. This change made it easier (at a lower cost) for the medical schools to discriminate against disfavored groups.[2]

Not surprisingly, the medical schools responded by discriminating against blacks, women, and Jews. Other disfavored ethnic and cultural groups suffered discrimination, but their plights have not been so well recorded. In 1910, seven black medical schools were operating. By 1930, only two remained. In 1910, 2.5 percent of physicians were black, and the percentage was increasing. After 1920, it fell continuously to 1.4 percent by 1969. After the medical schools were scaled down, some schools began to prohibit women completely, and many others enforced quotas limiting women to 5 percent of the student body (Starr 1982, 124). A peak in the proportion of women in medicine occurred in 1910 (Frech 1974, 124) and was not surpassed until recently.

---

1. For a detailed analysis of the history of licensure and professional restrictions in Ohio, see Lippincott (1982).

2. See Glen Cain (1986) or Donahue and Heckman (1991) for surveys of the literature on discrimination. See Gary Becker (1971) for the classic economic analysis of discrimination.

Discrimination against Jews was even more striking. It was often accomplished through explicit quotas. The dean of the Cornell Medical College in New York City, for example, explained in a 1940 letter that "Cornell Medical College admits a class of eighty each fall . . . from about twelve hundred applicants of whom seven hundred or more are Jews. We limit the (proportion) of Jews admitted to each class to from 10–15 percent" (Frech 1974, 125). Thus, a Jew had one chance in seventy of admission, while a gentile had one chance in seven.

During the depression, demand for medical care and physician incomes declined sharply. In response, the AMA and the state licensing boards successfully pressured the medical schools to reduce enrollments (Hyde and staff 1954, 971–73). While total enrollments were cut by 13 percent, the percentage of predominantly Jewish City College of New York applicants admitted to medical school anywhere in the country declined from 58 percent in 1925 to 15 percent in 1943 (Frech 1974, 126). Reuben Kessel argues that Jews bore the brunt of discrimination because they were culturally different, were suspicious of cartels and guilds, and thus were more likely to be competitive (1958, 46, 47).

Public Interest versus Monopoly in Theories of Licensure

Two major theories explain the history of occupational licensure found in the economics literature. The public interest theory holds that licensure serves the public interest by keeping fraudulent and incompetent sellers out of the market. The special interest, or monopoly, theory, conversely, argues that licensure is a monopolistic device whereby the government enforces a cartel.

The two theories of licensure are not mutually exclusive. No one's motives are likely to be purely altruistic or purely selfish. Further, it is possible that licensure, even if pursued entirely for selfish gain, nonetheless benefits the public.

Which Occupations Become Licensed. Two classic empirical studies of the origins of occupational licensure were done by Thomas Moore (1961) and by George Stigler (1971). Both used two models of licensure: the public interest, or idealistic, theory and the professional monopoly model. Both used the year of licensure in a state as a proxy for the strength of the licensure political movement. Moore found the earliness of licensure to be positively related to the total income and educational level of the occupation. He interpreted this as a proxy for the complexity and importance of the service provided and thus the public interest in regulating quality by licensure. Moore believed that this causation supports the public interest theory of licensure.

Stigler, in contrast, found the same earliness of licensure measure to be positively related to the relative size of the occupational group and urbanization. Taking these as proxies for the political power of the occupations themselves, he interpreted his results as supporting the professional monopoly model of licensure. Further, he compared the occupations across states and found that where they are licensed, the occupations were more stable in membership and had higher incomes, again proxies for the professions' political power.

Licensed occupations also tend to be self-employed, so that there is no organized political opposition to licensure by employers. But the quality-certifying function is likely also to be more important for self-employed professionals. Consumers have poorer information about quality than employers. Thus, this result is consistent with both views of licensure. Stigler also found that occupations with footloose employers, who could avoid any state's licensure by moving to other states, were less likely to be licensed. This finding supports his view.

Stigler's statistical comparisons of the same occupation across states with and without licensure are plagued with ambiguity about causation. Some of the characteristics are caused by licensure, not the other way around. Greater stability and higher incomes are clear examples. In principle, this flaw could be avoided by simultaneous equations methods if there were enough data. The variation in licensure over time and across states enables one, in principle, to identify the causal role of the occupations' characteristics.

Elizabeth Graddy (1991a, b) performed similar studies to test the two theories of licensure. In both studies she ran regressions across states to determine whether an occupation would be licensed. In one study, she examined six health occupations; in another, six occupations, two in health care. In both cases Graddy interpreted her results as supporting both the public interest and special interest theories. She found a positive relationship between clients being individuals and high education with licensure. Following Moore, she took this as evidence for the public interest theory. Unfortunately these relationships just as easily support the special-interest theories.

James Begun and Roger Feldman (1990) discussed the continued political appeal of licensure in the face of criticism by many scholars. They attribute support for licensure to fear and ignorance on the part of the general public. For the case of optometrists, they presented evidence against the public interest theory of licensure.

More research on licensure would be useful. Although the facts about licensing professions are clear, an interpretation of the reasoning is not.

Licensure, Information, and Certification. Consumers know that all licensed practitioners have met some minimum requirements. The costs of licensure include restriction of supply, possibly inappropriate education and preparation, and possible use of the licensing mechanism to restrict competition within the profession. Most costs of licensure follow from its mandatory nature. But there is an alternative in which professionals are certified as exceeding minimum standards but others are still allowed to practice.

This alternative is called certification, or, somewhat confusingly, permissive or voluntary licensure. This system provides as much information about the certified individuals as does licensure, without eliminating competition from uncertified individuals. Thus, it provides most of the benefits of licensure without most of the costs. Certification is common in the economy. Sometimes it is private, as in the Good Housekeeping seal, Underwriters Laboratories approval, or ratings by Consumers Union or the American Society of Anesthesiologists.

Though certification avoids some supply-reducing effects of licensure, certification itself can be manipulated to harm competition and earn monopoly rents (Havighurst 1984). The American College of Surgeons, for example, prohibits so-called itinerant practice whereby a surgeon leaves the postoperative care to a physician who is not a surgeon. This rule raises demand for surgeons. Dr. Robert Keofoot of Nebraska was recently ejected from the College of Surgeons because of this practice. With the help of the American Academy of Family Physicians, he (unsuccessfully) sued the college over this rule (Green 1987).

Yet, information used for consumer choice is a pure public good. Once produced and published, that knowledge can be used by any number of consumers: nothing efficiently prevents a consumer from passing such information along—an inherent difficulty in charging for the information. Thus, the main incentive to provide the information is to raise demand for some sellers. This is equally true for advertising and for certification of quality.

The main incentive for specialty and paramedical organizations to certify their members is to increase the public's demand for their services at the expense of uncertified practitioners. Such an incentive can lead certifying organizations to overstate the value of the certification and to be excessively strict—and thereby reduce the number of new certified practitioners who compete with existing certified members. Conversely, if existing certifiers are considered too restrictive, there may be incentives for competing certifying groups to emerge; two competing groups certify scuba diving. But scale economies may make entry difficult, especially into public certification. Thus, there is a role for judicial scrutiny to avoid the anticompetitive dangers of certification.

Oddly enough, one benefit of licensure requires that it confer monopoly rents on physicians. Benjamin Klein and Keith Leffler (1981) showed that the prospect of continued supracompetitive prices and monopoly rents encourages a supply of high-quality goods and services, even if consumers cannot detect quality until after purchase. In making a quality decision, the seller compares the future streams of rents, depending on whether he provides high or low quality. Low quality gives higher immediate profits but lower future profits when consumers learn about the low quality, and the seller's reputation suffers. High quality gives lower immediate profits but protects the ability to earn higher profits in the future. In this view, the monopoly return might be necessary to have the high-quality goods or services available in the market at all.

Although not mentioned by Klein and Leffler, the analysis applies directly to licensed professionals such as physicians (Svorney 1987, 499–502). Licensure ensures them high monopoly rents as long as they practice medicine.[3] The threat of losing their good reputations with fellow physicians and consumers is a powerful incentive for physicians to deliver high-quality services.[4] This function of licensure is independent of the criteria for licensure. Licenses could simply be sold to the

---

3. The application of the Klein and Leffler theory to individuals involves a slight technical problem because individuals have finite lives. Thus, using their model with the usual assumption of narrow rationality at all times, the incentives for high quality would unravel. An elegant proof of this proposition was developed by Duncan Luce and Howard Raiffa (1957). The implications of this theory of finite games are usually falsified experimentally (for example, Lave 1962). Also, many types of behavior (for example, collusion and even exchange) cannot be explained by narrow rationality and finite horizons. Thus, it seems necessary to abandon this model for many economic interactions, including the quality choices of individual physicians (Comanor and Frech 1987).

4. Perhaps showing the weakness of the consumer protection rationale for licensure, licensing boards rarely discipline errant or low-quality physicians, much less do they revoke licenses. In 1984, there were only 3.18 disciplinary actions taken per thousand physicians, and only 0.59 licenses revoked (Svorney 1987, 502). Further, sociological studies report that professional self-regulation does not protect the consumer from low-quality services (Huag 1980, 70–71).

highest bidder, as they might be in a corrupt system.

Similarly, Hayne Leland (1979) has shown that in some markets licensure with random selection can improve economic efficiency and consumer welfare: higher prices attract higher-quality sellers and consumers are totally and permanently ignorant of quality. The latter assumption seems particularly troublesome, but some version of his theoretical result probably follows even if that assumption is weakened.

Quality. One version of the idealistic theory of licensure holds that licensure is necessary because the quality of care without it would be unacceptably low. There are two possible interpretations of this statement. One holds that, absent licensure, consumers would be fooled into buying lower-quality services than they prefer. This view simply restates the idea that licensure provides valuable information. Certification could provide the same information with fewer monopolistic side effects.

The alternative interpretation holds that even with perfect information, consumers would choose services of too low a quality. This authoritarian, or paternalistic, position differs from the informational view. Licensure may not raise overall quality.

Early licensure and quality. The claim that actual physician licensure in the eighteenth and nineteenth centuries raised quality was, in retrospect, laughable. For hundreds of years, the so-called scientific physicians, the forerunners of today's doctors, were treating their patients by bloodletting, applying cathartics, and poisoning. Surgeons knew nothing of cleanliness. Richard Shryock, a distinguished medical historian, argued (1967) that one's health was harmed, not helped, by physicians until the early twentieth century. The followers of herbal medicine, homeopathy, and so on opposed the heroic measures and therefore did less harm to their patients. Early licensure, to the extent that it did anything, reduced the average quality of physician services as it raised its cost.

Today medical care is clearly beneficial to health—at least most of the time. But the medical profession is still shockingly ignorant of the actual effects of many of its medicines and procedures. Millions of women, for example, were given diethylstilbestrol (DES) for problems of pregnancy. Their daughters are more prone to cancer than the average of the population; at the time the drug companies or doctors could not have known this effect of DES. Yet, the scientific community knew that DES did not actually help in pregnancy. Another excellent example is the internal mammary ligation, tying off the mammary arteries to divert blood to the heart—supposedly a cure for coronary artery disease. Hundreds of thousands of these operations were performed before some small-scale studies showed it to be useless (Spodick 1985, 117, 122).

To make scientifically rational choices of drugs, physicians must compare costs and effectiveness. Yet, in his excellent study of drug regulation, Peter Temin (1980) found little scientific knowledge of the comparative effectiveness of different drugs because the necessary research has not been undertaken. The biochemical mechanism of how most drugs work is unknown. Further, what limited information exists on comparative effectiveness is typically ignored by physicians.

Studies of doctors' actual prescribing behavior have shown it to be conventional, based on medical customs. Most studies compared prescribing behavior to customs or norms, such as avoiding the antibiotic chloramphenicol. That particular norm seems irrational since the mortality risk of the drug is low, lower than penicillin. Temin argued that using chloramphenicol is not necessarily a prescribing error (1980, 95, 110). He concluded that (1980, 119) "doctors cannot and do not make informed choices among competing drugs."

The scientific medicine supposedly enshrined by modern licensure is not so scientific after all. It has its own traditions and conventions that have not been studied. Even so, it might seem that licensure, by preventing entry of those with poorer academic backgrounds, improves quality. Yet, that may not be so. The quality of the average physician has risen. But consumers' substitution of other services such as chiropractors, self-care, and the advice of friends plus physician substitution of nurses and technicians for their own time may have reduced the quality of the care actually received. Michael Pertschuk, former chairman of the Federal Trade Commission, noted that the highest death rate from electrocution occurred in states with the most restrictive systems for licensing electricians (1980, 346). For physicians, this case was forcefully made by a New Jersey hospital administrator opposing restrictions on foreign-trained physicians (Stevens and Vermeulen 1971, III-8):

> It's easy to sit behind a desk in Chicago (the headquarters of the American Medical Association) and frame ideals about the quality of care. But, a supposedly non-qualified doctor can put on a tourniquet and give the usual drugs and plasma for shock to tide the patient over . . . And that's better than having the patient die.

Studies of licensure and quality. There have been several studies of the effect of licensure on quality of services. Pertschuk (1980, 345–46) noted that several FTC studies of licensure and quality showed little or no relationship. Conversely, Alex Maurizi (1980) found that the quality of California contractors, at least as measured by the ratio of complaints to licensees, declined as the licensing examination became easier to pass. Unfortunately, this is a poor measure of quality and is likely to be responsive to the increase in publicity for the consumers' movement, which coincided with the easing of the contractor's examination. If raising quality is the main motive behind licensure, one must ask: Why are there no requirements for periodical retesting? After all, that is common for drivers and pilots.

Recent Challenges to the Standard View. The mainstream view among economists who have studied physician licensure follows Kessel's classic (1958) article. Based on the history of licensure, it holds that organized medicine used licensure, as well as control of the medical schools, to restrict entry and to raise the monopoly rents of the profession (Kessel 1958; Friedman and Kuznets 1954; Friedman 1962; Rayack 1967; Frech 1974; Feldstein 1977, 57–60).

Keith Leffler (1978), Thomas Hall and Matt Lindsay (1980), and Leffler and Lindsay (1981) have subsequently challenged that view. Those authors were not greatly concerned with the actual history of the licensure movement or the motives of the participants. Instead, they looked to statistical measures of the behavior of licensure across space and over time. Thus, they took the same approach as Moore, Stigler, and Graddy, discussed above. Leffler found that variation in the difficulty of licensure across states was correlated with proxies for the demand for quality certification, such as the percentage of poor and old and the stability of the population (1978, 180–83). But such a procedure does not distinguish between the two theories of licensure. Politics constrains even a perfectly monopolistic licensure movement, so Leffler's variables may reflect interstate variation in the political constraints the licensed industries felt.

Some of Leffler's other findings are not consistent with the consumer information theory of licensure. He found that a state exemption of physicians who have passed the national board exam could not be explained by the public's interest in quality assurance. The states not accepting the national board exam did not have high demand for quality certification. Further, physician's incomes were higher in those states (1978, 184–85). Chris Paul (1982) found that the political structure of state medical licensing boards was related to physicians' incomes. Where the medical society selects the board members, physicians' incomes are higher. In dentistry Deborah Freund and Jay

61

Schulman (1984) found strong evidence that state examinations created entry barriers.

Hall and Lindsay (1980) took a different tack. They estimated a noncollusive model for individual medical school output over the period 1959 to 1973. The model explains variation in enrollment and tuition over the period based on applicant demand for positions, donations for medical education, and costs. They believe that those findings contradict the traditional view that organized medicine has influenced medical schools to reduce the supply of physicians. But their interpretation is false.

No one argues that the AMA and the medical schools are a perfect cartel. Rather, the traditional claim is that the AMA influenced state licensing boards to require AMA certification of medical schools and raised the standards for medical school accreditation to reduce the supply of medical education, and therefore of physicians. Medical schools are accredited for a fixed number of students, a practice unknown in disciplines without licensure (Noether 1986, 233). Having lost a considerable amount of political power since World War II, the AMA's control over individual schools' enrollment is now weaker (Noether 1986, 233–35).

Political and economic processes constrain organized medicine. When demand for medical care increases, it would be rational for organized medicine, even if it had perfect control of medical training, to raise enrollments. Hall and Lindsay found that medical school enrollment responded to demand for medical care. That does not even disprove an extreme perfect collusion version of the traditional understanding.

The work of Leffler and Lindsay (1981) is closely related. Using aggregate national data, they estimated a simple supply and demand model for physicians. They explained a good deal of the variation over time in physicians' incomes and numbers with their straightforward approach. But the fact that competitive models fit the data is not evidence that the market is competitive. The opposite does not follow either. Economic theory shows that the poor statistical performance of a competitive model is not evidence that the market is not competitive.

Monopolistic and competitive markets respond to external shocks in about the same way. Consider an increase in demand. In a competitive market where supply is an increasing function of price, the result would be higher price and higher output. A monopolist would also raise price and output, unless the new higher demand curve were much more elastic (flatter). If the demand elasticities are stable or are related to observed variables (for example, insurance coverage), the competitive model will fit the data well, even when the market is actually monopolistic (Frech and Ginsburg 1972). Supply and demand models applied to market data cannot distinguish between competition and monopoly.

Shirley Svorney (1987) has taken a novel approach to testing whether current physician licensure is in consumers' interest. She argues that more restrictive licensure would raise or lower the equilibrium quantity of medical care, depending on whether the extra restrictions were in consumers' interests. If the restrictions were worth their cost to consumers, they would raise demand for physician care by more than their costs. If they benefited consumers, the extra restrictions should be associated with higher quantity of physician care. If they harmed consumers but benefited physicians, the extra restrictions should be associated with lower use of physician services.

Svorney used 1965 data to avoid the confusing effects of the large immigration of foreign medical graduates since then. She found that two restrictions, a basic science certificate and a citizenship requirement, were associated with fewer physicians' services at the 95 percent level of significance. Thus, these extra restrictions harmed consumers and benefited physicians.

Since about 1890, the U.S. organized medical profession has succeeded in limiting entry. But since World War II, it has lost important political battles over the supply of physicians. In the 1960s, state and federal programs designed to expand medical school enrollment were enacted. Simultaneously immigration restrictions on and state licensure requirements for foreign medical graduates were relaxed, especially during the 1960s and 1970s (Noether 1986, 233–43). From 1960 to 1983, the number of medical schools rose from 91 to 142, and the number of physicians per 100,000 population from 151 to 228. From 1970 to 1983, the number of foreign medical graduates rose from 54,000 to 100,000 (U.S. Bureau of the Census 1990, 101). Noether estimated that monopoly rents of physicians had declined from 30 percent of their income in 1972 to 20 percent in 1982 (1986, 233).

Supply Restriction in Dentistry

The history of supply restriction in dentistry closely followed that of physicians. In 1834, the first dental society, the New York Society of Surgeon Dentists, tried to stop the spread of what it called quackery (the use of the new, less painful amalgam metal in fillings). In 1840, the American Society of Dental Surgeons was founded to restrict entry and to oppose the use of amalgam. The society tried to force states to pass licensure laws, but its timing was poor. At the height of the Jacksonian antimonopoly movement, the states were busy repealing whatever licensure laws they already had, not passing new ones. The society folded in 1856 over the amalgam issue. Many regular dentists, including some society members, had adopted the new metal (which is now the standard material for fillings).

By the late 1800s, the dental associations had succeeded in persuading many states to adopt licensure that the associations themselves controlled. Just as in medicine, licensure required a dental school diploma. The immediate result was rapid entry of new dental schools and no slowing of the entry of new dentists.

Following the 1926 publication of the Gies report, *Dental Education in the United States and Canada,* paralleling the Flexner report for medicine, entry was restricted (Feldstein 1988, 89). The dental practice acts were amended to require an examination and graduation from an approved dental school. The state boards of dental examiners, controlled by the dental societies, gained the power to approve dental schools. As a result, the number of dental schools and students rapidly declined (Fraundorf 1984, 759–73).

Interestingly, one of the standards was that the schools could not be profit-seeking, regardless of their actual quality. Although the dental societies claimed that the profit-seeking schools thus eliminated had been turning out below-par dentists, a statistical study showed that graduates of some profit-seeking schools had better pass rates on the examinations than the graduates of the top-rated nonprofit schools (Fraundorf 1984, 731). Also paralleling the case of physicians, organized dentistry has lost political power in recent years, and entry into dentistry has increased. From 1960 to 1984, the number of dental schools rose from forty-seven to sixty, and the number of dentists per 100,000 population from 47 to 57 (U.S. Bureau of the Census 1987, 90).

In dentistry, restrictions on the method of practice that reduce the output per dentist have been more important than in medicine. In particular, there are severe restrictions on the use of dental assistants and hygienists and on the number of offices that a dentist can operate. These restrictions are imposed at the state level and vary across states. Cross-sectional statistical analyses show that these restrictions raise the prices of dental care and the incomes of dentists (Liang and Ogur 1987).

Organized Medicine and Competition within the Profession

While the actions of organized physicians have reduced entry into medicine, they have also reduced competition among those who may enter. The attempts to reduce internal competition have a long history.

Price Fixing. The first known example of price fixing was in the colony of New Jersey. The New Jersey Medical Society's first official act in 1766 created a table of minimum fees, called a fee bill. Members were to be expelled for charging lower prices (Berlant 1981, 8; Blumberg 1984, 328). The Boston Medical Society promulgated a fee bill sometime before 1787 (Blumberg 1984, 304–5). Local societies established minimum fees in Charleston and New York City before 1800.

Local price fixing subsequently became more common. The first AMA code of ethics, adopted in 1847, urged price fixing by local medical societies in every community (Konold 1962, 11). The 1903 revision of the code of ethics suggested that the fees agreed on by the local medical societies be considered minimums, preserving the right of physicians to charge more (Berlant 1975, 101). By 1850, price fixing was common in large cities. By 1910, fee bills were also common in small towns (Konold 1962, 2, 56). In 1906, the AMA denounced an attempt by life insurers to pay $3, rather than the previous $5, for examinations and forbade members to perform examinations for less than $5. The AMA was successful, and the insurers backed down (Konold 1962, 57).

The attempts to fix prices sometimes generated active consumer opposition. When the Medical Association of the District of Columbia fixed fees in 1833, aggrieved consumers held protest meetings and offered support and protection for out-of-town physicians to settle in Washington (Konold 1962, 7). In 1902, the physician who had been AMA president in 1899 wrote that "the most despicable character is the one who starts in to undercharge his competitors in order to advance his number of patients" (Berlant 1975, 100).

In the 1912 revision of the code of ethics, the AMA rejected a clause renewing support for local fee setting. Apparently, the idea was to encourage price discrimination, charging higher prices to those who were more willing and able to pay (Kessel 1958). In 1957, fees reappeared in the code of ethics, which encouraged fees commensurate with the patient's ability to pay (Berlant 1975, 104).

Since the 1975 Supreme Court decision in *Goldfarb v. Virginia State Bar Association*, collective fee setting by professional associations has been clearly illegal. Other activities that influence fees directly, such as the promulgation of relative fee schedules, have also been under antitrust attack.

Relative Value Scales. In contrast to much professional society activity that is designed to reduce consumer information, relative value scales (RVSs) improve market information. RVSs simplify the pricing of physician services and the determination of insurance benefits. RVSs assign each procedure a number that represents its relative value or relative price. To arrive at the actual dollar price, the number from the scale must be multiplied by the conversion factor. An RVS, for example, might assign 50 to a tonsillectomy and 110 to an appendectomy. A physician using the RVSs would multiply each number by a conversion factor, say $10 per unit, to arrive at the actual fee to be charged, $500 and $1,100. To use the RVS to define insurance benefits, an insurer would select a conversion factor to arrive at the maximum benefit it would pay for each procedure.

Rvss are a modern phenomenon. Except for Medicare's new system, all RVSs have been developed by physician associations. The California Medical Society promulgated the first one in 1956. The AMA endorsed RVSs in 1958. Many other state medical societies have developed RVSs, as have specialist societies. Many state societies have endorsed RVSs developed elsewhere, especially California's. Some insurers use RVSs as the basis of their reimbursement (Havighurst and Kissam 1979, 48–50).

Antitrust authorities have widely attacked RVSs for improving doctors' information about competitors' prices and thus facilitating explicit or tacit collusion. Generally, professional societies have agreed to stop promulgating the indexes without going to court. Examples include the American College of Obstetricians and Gynecologists, the American Academy of Orthopaedic Surgeons, the American College of Radiology, the Minnesota State Medical Association, the California Medical Association, and the Illinois Podiatry Association (Havighurst and Kissam 1979, 78). Surprisingly the Justice Department lost the one case that has been litigated (*United States v. the American Society of Anesthesiologists* 1979).

Dangers of RVSs. An RVS improves the information that physicians have about the pricing behavior of their competitors and thus eases concerted pricing and detection of price-cutters. It is a well-known principle that improving the information that sellers have about each other can reduce competition. This was the key of the Federal Trade Commission's and the Justice Department's objection to the professional societies' RVSs.

There is evidence that RVSs were sometimes used by societies to try to raise prices. The FTC found that the conversion factor to be used was discussed at county medical society meetings in Minnesota. One physician, somewhat confused about the meaning of competition, complained to the FTC that the local Blue Shield plan was violating the antitrust laws by choosing a lower conversion factor than his medical society had agreed on. The 1962 RVS from the American Society of Anesthesiologists included an explicit statement that it was intended to help local societies construct fee schedules (Havighurst and Kissam 1979, 52, 54, 55).

Even without explicit agreement on a conversion factor and thus prices, RVSs can discourage price competition and enhance price discrimination. An RVS can be used to raise the price of services that are the focus of price competition by assigning them a high value. Thus, a physician who desires to compete by price must either deviate from the RVS to reduce price only for the visible service or cut his price on all the services. Either way, the RVS has made price competition less attractive.

Competition focusing on visible services reduces their prices below what would be ideal from the viewpoint of the profession as a monopoly. Thus, an RVS that can raise the relative price of these services, even if it did nothing else, would raise the income of the physicians. At least one RVS was designed with this in mind. In 1971, the RVS of the American College of Obstetricians and Gynecologists was revised to raise the relative price of total pregnancy service to at least the value of a hysterectomy (Havighurst and Kissam, 1979, 57). Total pregnancy service is a good example of a well-defined, well-understood service that is a focus of price competition.

Benefits of RVSs. The RVS is a double-edged sword. Just as the information provided to physicians about their competitor's pricing tends to reduce competition, the information provided to consumers and their insurance companies tends to enhance competition. Where an RVS is used, consumers need know only a single price to determine which physicians are charging more. This knowledge eases the search and makes the market more competitive. Similarly, insurers can use the RVS as a simple way to state the maximum prices they will pay under fee schedule systems. Even under other insurance systems, widespread use of RVSs reduces the dispersion of prices. Therefore, the insurer learns more about a physician's pricing policies from a smaller sample of prices. This system can be used in a review of prices for reasonableness, negotiations with individual physicians, or in PPOs for selection of preferred providers.

Rickard Pfizenmayer (1982) defended RVSs on the novel ground that they simplify collective bargaining between organized physicians and the third-party payers. While RVSs may serve this function, this defense amounts to an admission that RVSs are anticompetitive; it is clearly anticompetitive for the physicians as a group to bargain about their fees. The antitrust laws were designed to prevent competitors from acting in concert to affect their prices, not to facilitate such practices.

Havighurst and Kissam (1979, 75, 76) argued that the benefits of RVSs could be obtained without harm to competition if the RVSs were produced by disinterested parties, not the doctors themselves. They suggested insurers for that task.

Empirical evidence on RVSs. Actual RVSs either decrease competition and raise prices or the reverse. Barry Eisenberg (1980) investigated this question with the AMA's data on physician fees. Using data on standard metropolitan statistical areas, he related the level and dispersion of fees to the use of RVSs. The use of RVSs varies across cities. Where RVSs were used, the price dispersion was far less. Going from no physicians using RVSs to all physicians using them cut the dispersion in half. This suggests better consumer information. The dispersion equations were interesting in other ways. As Pauly and Satterthwaite (1981) predicted, in SMSAs with more physicians per capita the price dispersion was wider.

Many have argued that group practices, being more visible than solo practices, would improve consumer information (Friedman 1962; Getzen 1984). This would tend to reduce price dispersion. Also, the prices within the group would typically be more uniform than prices across the market as a whole. For both reasons, one would expect that a larger average size of practice would lower price dispersion.

Conversely, group practices flourish in cities where the information is poor, as shown by Thomas Getzen (1984). Poorer information, thus larger price dispersion, would cause more physicians to select group practice. Theoretically, one cannot say which direction of causation would dominate. Empirically, the average size of practice and the price dispersion were positively correlated. Further research to determine the causation of group practice growth would be fruitful.

On the average level of fees, the key antitrust concern, the data were not helpful. The use of RVSs was faintly positively related to average fee, but for the three fees studied, the t statistics ranged from 0.84 to -0.14. The point estimates for the dollar effect of the RVS on initial office visit, follow-up office visit, and follow-up hospital visit are 2.7, 0.41 and -0.0051 (Eisenberg 1980, 455). Because the 2.7 estimate is about 10 to 15 percent of the mean fees, a precise estimate would be economically meaningful if it were estimated with precision. But such weak results are simply not informative.

The anesthesiologists' RVS case. In *United States v. the American Society of Anesthesiologists,* in 1979, the court found that the development of the relative value scale helped the insurers to establish a rational basis for reimbursing anesthesiologists. The court stressed that the insurers asked the American Society of Anesthesiologists to develop an

RVS for such use. Despite the RVS's explicit encouragement of local fee schedules, the court found that the society never encouraged the setting of common conversion factors. The court even endorsed collective negotiation of allowed fees between organized physician groups and insurers (Pfizenmayer 1982, 130–35).

This decision is bizarre since groups of physicians do not have the labor union exemption to the antitrust laws. Havighurst and Kissam (1979, 70) noted that "collective bargaining by the organized profession over third parties' approach to reimbursement offends basic antitrust principles." While the judge's decision that the anesthesiologists' RVS did not harm competition may be correct, his reasoning was not.

Opposition to Contract Medicine and HMOs. Contract medicine was an early precursor of the contemporary HMO. Under these plans, a physician would contract to provide all necessary medical care in return for a fixed annual sum. Contract medicine's incentives are identical to HMOs'. The risk is borne by the providers. The plans were formed by all sorts of groups, such as fraternal organizations and lodges, railroads, logging, mining and, less often, manufacturing firms. Some were formed by laymen for the sole purpose of obtaining medical insurance and care. Such plans were most popular among urban laborers. Spotty evidence suggests contract medicine was common.

Contract medicine was practiced in Boston as early as 1721 (Blumberg 1984, 323, n. 48). In New Orleans, an estimated 80 percent of the population was covered in 1888; 41 percent of the orthodox physicians participated in contract practice. At one point, the average annual fee was bid down to 40 cents per person (Berlant 1975, 254–55). Contract practice continued into the twentieth century. A survey of 100 cities in 1903 estimated that 3 percent of the population was covered by contract through lodges and fraternal orders alone (Konold 1962, 58). A contract between the Union Pacific Railroad and the Eugene (Oregon) Clinic survived into the 1970s.

Organized medicine opposed contract medicine from the beginning. Contract medicine was banned by the Georgia Medical Society of Savannah in 1807 and by the Boston Medical Association in 1808–1809 (Blumberg 1984, 323). The AMA classified it as unethical as early as 1869 but had little means to stop it. Physicians opposed such contracting because it provided a mechanism for price competition by bidding. The AMA approved contract practice where the physician's regular rates would be paid, but obtaining a discount was one of the purposes of contract practice (Konold 1962, 57–58).

Opposition to the modern forms of contract medicine, the HMO and the PPO, continues (Havighurst 1978, 316–19; *Medical Staff of Doc-*

tors' Hospital of Prince Georges County 1988). Group practice per se was disparaged as unethical as late as 1950. Since then, opposition has concentrated on groups that provide prepaid care (Hyde and staff 1954, 977–78). Opposition to PPOs primarily takes the form of lobbying state legislatures to pass laws harmful to them. Modern lobbying, mostly by state medical and hospital associations, has successfully added to barriers to PPOs in some states (Lindsey 1986; Winslow 1991).

Methods of opposition. Organized physicians have used many methods to slow the growth of HMOs. Most methods involve denial of membership applications or expulsion by the local county medical societies. A network of legal and informal relationships among the AMA, hospitals, malpractice insurers, speciality boards, state licensing boards, and even the U.S. Navy reinforces the importance of medical society membership.

In the past, membership in the local medical society was a prerequisite for hospital privileges at many hospitals. The Mundt resolution, passed by the AMA House of Delegates in 1934, required that a hospital's medical staff be members of their local medical society for that hospital to be accredited for internship training by the AMA. This accreditation was required by state licensing boards and speciality boards. Unaccredited hospitals were cut off from a lucrative source of cheap labor. This rule affected most hospitals, representing as much as 99 percent of a state's hospital beds (Hyde and staff 1954, 952–53).

Many specialty boards, as well, required membership in the county society. Nonmembers often found it difficult to obtain malpractice insurance, either because the local or state medical society sold the insurance itself or because commercial insurers charged a higher price to nonmembers. The latter was rational since it was easier for malpractice plaintiffs to get local physicians to testify against nonmembers. Some nonmembers were forced to go to Lloyds of London for their malpractice insurance (Hyde and staff 1954; 951).

Some states required that an out-of-state physician be a member of the medical society of his home state. During World War II, the U.S. Navy required the same. If a member's conduct was found to be unethical by a local medical society, for example, by working for an HMO, other members were forbidden to associate with him under pain of expulsion (Hyde and staff 1954, 962).

Local medical societies used these weapons against the closed panel prepaid group practices, the early HMOs. A well-known early episode concerned the Group Health Association of Washington, D.C. The organization violated the AMA's code of ethics in several ways. First, the physicians were paid a salary. Second, the plan was controlled by laymen. Most important, the plan restricted choice to a closed panel of physicians. The District of Columbia Medical Society expelled or disciplined many of the doctors involved. Some physicians were induced by the threat of expulsion to resign from GHA. The society prohibited its members from associating with GHA physicians. The District Society enlisted the help of the AMA to deny GHA physicians staff privileges at D.C. hospitals. The final result was a successful criminal prosecution of the AMA by the Justice Department for antitrust violations (*American Medical Association* 1943). Havighurst (1978), Barton (1974), and Kessel (1958) provide excellent accounts of other battles against HMOs.

While professional opposition to HMOs may be more subtle and harder to discover now, it continues. In the mid-1980s, the Federal Trade Commission charged a group of doctors in suburban Washington, D.C., with trying to prevent Health Plan, the HMO of George Washington University Medical School faculty, from setting up shop. Among other legal complaints, the physicians were accused of threatening to boycott and thus to shut down a local hospital if it helped the HMO to open a clinic (*Medical Staff of Doctor's Hospital of Prince Georges County* 1988).

The organized medical profession has also opposed insurer cost controls that are milder than those of the typical HMO. Lawrence Goldberg and Warren Greenberg (1977a) reviewed an antitrust suit brought against the Oregon State Medical Society. They found that as early as the 1920s, the Oregon insurers used modern cost-containment techniques, such as prior approval for hospitalization. These techniques were finally dropped because of the concerted opposition of the medical profession and especially the medical society's sponsorship of Oregon Blue Shield. In the early 1980s, the Michigan State Medical Society boycotted Blue Shield to force it to drop a cost-control program. After investigation, the FTC issued a cease-and-desist order (1983) against the medical society.

Physician Networks and the Antitrust Guidelines. The fear that physician groups might oppose HMO and PPO medicine, or more likely raise their fees under it, continues to inform modern antitrust policy. In late 1994, American antitrust enforcement agencies issued a joint document on principles for health care markets (U.S. Department of Justice and the Federal Trade Commission 1994). The section on physician network joint ventures (statement 8, 66–88) has generated continuing controversy and criticism.

The enforcement agencies have taken the position that independent physicians cannot organize merely for the purpose of negotiating prices. This action would amount to price fixing and therefore be illegal per se. The situation also might undermine the growth of HMOs and PPOs generally. Therefore, physician organizations must have some other purpose, such as risk sharing for providing a new product. There have already been two antitrust consent decrees following this policy in 1995 (Raskin, n.d.).

The other viewpoint, taken by Clark Havighurst (1995), Richard Raskin (n.d.), and others, is that physician organizations may reduce the transactions costs involved in setting up competing managed care systems. Therefore, they should not be considered illegal per se. Physician networks that are limited solely to joint selling may be both procompetitive and proefficiency.

Hospital Access. Sometimes entire classes of physicians are simply not given hospital privileges. This exclusion is probably most often directed against doctors of osteopathy.[5] Such action was judged anticompetitive in the landmark 1984 antitrust case of *Weiss v. York Hospital,* which is analyzed in Frech (1985). Out-of-town physicians are sometimes excluded by residency requirements. This type of blanket exclusion usually requires the cooperation of the entire medical staff of a hospital but generally runs counter to the economic interest of the hospital itself. The hospital ordinarily is better off with a larger medical staff to raise demand.

On a smaller scale, individual physicians or physician groups may sometimes obtain exclusive contracts to provide particular services in a hospital and by so doing exclude other physicians from using the facilities. This is especially common in the most hospital-oriented services: radiology, pathology, and anesthesiology. While these exclusive contracts reduce competition, there also may be efficiency advantages. William Lynk and Michael Morrisey (1987) maintained that physicians can more efficiently share in the management of facilities if they must perform all their practice in a single hospital. They conducted an empirical analysis relating the use of exclusive contracts to concentration in the local market and found a slight negative relation. Lynk and Mor-

---

5. Founded in the nineteenth century, osteopathy originally focused on manipulation of the spine, much like chiropracty. Along with chiropracty, it was attacked by the AMA as quackery. In the early twentieth century, however, osteopathic training and practice evolved to the point of being indistinguishable from orthodox medicine. By midcentury, the AMA had rescinded its condemnation of osteopathy, and osteopathic physicians had achieved identical legal rights of practice. Osteopaths are now found in all branches of federal government service.

rissey interpreted this as evidence that the exclusive contracts do not give market power to physicians. But their data show that exclusive contracts are common even in local areas with a single monopoly hospital. That none of the efficiency arguments seem to hold in such situations lends credence to a market power explanation.

Other Restrictions. Organized physicians have attempted to prevent competition in other ways. As far back as Hippocrates, ethical codes have generally prohibited advertising and opposed both price and quality competition. Early ethical rules in England prohibited public criticism of a fellow physician, an idea that has continued in the United States. The 1543 statutes of the Royal College of Physicians prohibited consulting with unlicensed physicians and providing information about medicines to the public (Berlant 1975, 84–85). The AMA's ethics show a similar approach. The first code of ethics, adopted in 1847, advised physicians to hide disagreements with each other from patients and to avoid public criticism of a fellow physician. The rules prohibited soliciting patients of another physician. Consulting with irregular practitioners (that is, those not approved by the AMA) was also prohibited.

The prohibition against consultation with irregular physicians was part of organized medicine's long-term opposition to what it called quackery. Although it now seems laughable, the idea that irregular medicine was unscientific was seriously promoted. During the nineteenth century, the definition of unorthodox practitioners was somehow stretched to cover women, no matter how orthodox their training and practices. Women were finally accepted by the turn of the century (Konold 1962, 23–24). Similar rules were used against black physicians. They were denied membership in local or state societies and thus kept out of white hospitals regardless of their training (Konold 1962, 24).

Beginning in 1903, the AMA opposed fee splitting, the practice of specialists sharing their fees with the physician from whom they received their referrals (Berlant 1975, 98, 99). Mark Pauly (1979) showed that fee splitting helped the market for specialists' services to become more competitive. The existence of fee splitting demonstrates that the specialists had market power, that their prices exceeded their marginal costs. Otherwise, there would be no rents available from which to pay the generalist who made the referral. Through fee splitting, specialists competed with each other. At least some benefits of this competition were passed on to consumers as lower prices for generalists. Prohibiting fee splitting thus insulates the specialists from competition and raises their incomes.

The incentives for fee splitting are strong since prices for the specialized service exceed marginal costs. Prohibitions on fee splitting are often circumvented by the integration of the referred service with the referring physician. This integration commonly happens by joint ownership in the multispeciality group practice, especially those with extensive capability for medical tests. Physicians also integrate by contract, whereby physicians operate joint ventures with hospitals or testing centers. This latter is opposed by Congress (especially in Medicare rules); the former goes generally unnoticed and unremarked.

Since competition and consumer information are imperfect, there are incentives for unethical referrals—those that are not in the patient's best interest. With fee splitting, there is a possible incentive for referrals to a specialist when it would be better for the generalist to perform the treatment. Without fee splitting, there is an incentive for the generalist to perform the work himself when a referral would be better for the patient. As Pauly observed, it is not obvious that the incentives for appropriate referrals are better without fee splitting. The incentives are better if the specialists' market is more competitive (Pauly 1979, 352).

Physician specialty groups sometimes try to impose rules that restrict competition from other specialties. These rules sometimes arouse opposition from other specialties. The American College of Surgeons, a specialty group, has a rule that a surgeon must do his own postoperative care. This rule is designed to reduce the output per surgeon and thus to restrict supply and maintain upward pressure on fees. Just as clearly, this rule reduces the demand for general or family practitioners and works hardships on patients in rural areas. As mentioned above, this rule has been unsuccessfully legally challenged by Dr. Robert Keofoot and the American Academy of Family Physicians (Green 1987).

The Degree of Competition among Physicians

As shown above, comparative static behavior cannot distinguish competition from monopoly. But some analyses can. First, let us be precise about the meanings of perfect competition and monopoly; I use the terms in the standard economic way.

Thus, I take monopoly to mean that each independent physician can raise his fees without losing any of his patients. His existing patients will each demand less of his services, but none will switch. Cross-elasticities of demand among physicians are zero. Under monopoly, each physician faces a fraction of the market demand curve, with the same price elasticity as that market demand curve. Each physician is economically isolated from substitute physicians. Another monopoly model would be based on perfect collusion among physicians.

The polar extreme is perfect competition. Under perfect competition, each physician is a price taker. He can sell all he wants at the going market rate and nothing at all if he sets his price slightly above that rate.

Competition Exists. Much evidence rejects the monopoly model of the physician market. The analysis is similar to that for hospital competition above.

Demand is too inelastic for monopoly. First, the monopoly model predicts that the individual physicians, therefore the entire market, would face price-elastic demand (where the demand is more price elastic than − 1.0). If sellers were to face a demand curve less elastic than this, they would raise revenue and reduce costs by raising prices. This situation would continue until the seller's price and quantity combination rose up his demand curve into the elastic region. There is much evidence that the market demand for both physician and hospital care is less price responsive than − 1.0. It is approximately − 0.2. If physicians were monopolists, either collectively or individually, the elasticity of demand facing them would be the same as the market elasticity and it would be greater (more negative) than − 1.0.

Selling below market prices and physician density. The monopoly model also predicts that physicians' willingness to serve consumers below market prices would be independent of the physician density. Under monopoly, there is no prospect of taking patients away from one's competitors, so it would not matter how many competitors there are. Yet, there is evidence from the Medicare program that physicians are more willing to accept assignment (that is, agree to treat patients for less than their customary fee) in metropolitan areas. In the early 1980s in Massachusetts, such assignment rates were 83 percent in Boston and 51 percent on mostly rural Cape Cod. For ophthalmology, the rates were 50 percent and 13 percent. John Larkin Thompson, president of Massachusetts Blue Shield, the Medicare carrier, attributes the difference to differences in competition. The metropolitan versus nonmetropolitan difference is found everywhere (Thompson 1983, 110, 112).

Price competition by accepting assignment is less demanding of consumer information than ordinary price competition. Simply telling the Medicare beneficiary that one accepts assignment conveys the necessary information. To aid competition further, several states and local private organizations have published lists of physicians who accept assignment for Medicare consumers. Insurance paying somewhat less than market, where physicians can compete by agreeing with consumers not to balance bill, encourages competition. At least for physician competition, Medicare has, perhaps accidentally, chosen a reasonable benefit structure. Unfortunately the growth of Medicare supplementary (Medigap) insurance since 1966 has progressively undermined the cost controls and procompetitive features of Medicare physician insurance.

Consumer choice of provider and insurance. The monopoly model also predicts that consumer choice of physician would not be affected by net price, therefore would not be affected by the type of insurance. Yet the available evidence shows that consumers with indemnity insurance choose lower-priced physicians and hospitals than those with co-insured benefits (Newhouse and Phelps 1974).[6] Consumers with the more complete Blue Cross coverage choose more costly hospitals (Andersen and Anderson 1970). In markets with higher hospital insurance coverage, the price of surgery is higher, with an elasticity of 0.15. Thus, an increase of average coinsurance from 0.80 to 0.88 would increase the price of surgery by 1.5 percent (Cromwell and Mitchell 1986, 303). This estimate is biased downward by measurement error in the insurance coverage variable since it is based on state data and applies to hospitalization, not surgery (see the discussion below). A recent paper by M. Susan Marquis (1985), based on a RAND experiment, finds little effect of insurance on choice of provider.

The difference between Marquis's experimental results and the earlier nonexperimental ones may be due to the short length of the experiment (three years) or to insufficiently deep cost sharing. Or perhaps altering the search incentives of one family, while not changing those of its network of friends and relatives, has less effect than altering the incentives of the entire group. Nonexperimental data would capture some effects of changing incentives for the whole recommending group. Or the problem may be important omitted variables. There is clearly a need for further research on the connection between insurance benefit structure and choice of provider.

Competition Is Not Perfect. At the other extreme is the model of perfect competition. It can be disproved almost as easily as the monopoly model.

---

6. As discussed above, indemnity insurance pays up to a fixed dollar amount per unit of service. It might pay, for example, $1,500 for an appendectomy. The consumer is responsible to pay for any extra, which is called the balance bill.

Selling below market prices. Perfectly competitive physicians would not treat consumers at below market prices since they could get as much business as they wanted at the going prices. Yet, in many programs physicians supply their services in return for fees below market rates. In the Medicaid program prices are typically set well below the market. The wealthy states of the Northeast are the most extreme in this regard. In 1979, New York, for example, paid specialists only 24 percent of the Medicare allowances, which was already about 25–30 percent below market. Pennsylvania paid only slightly better, at 29 percent. The most generous states in the Northeast, Vermont and New Hampshire, paid only 68 percent of Medicare's allowances (Holahan 1984). The discounts are almost as deep for general practitioners. Despite these deep discounts, some physicians (not all) treat Medicaid patients.

During the era of free pricing, before 1991, Medicare allowances were about 25–30 percent below market, yet about 80 percent of physicians accepted assignment. No doubt some Medicare enrollees received a lower quality product as the physician spent less time and effort because of the lower prices, but in many specialties the possibilities for quality adjustment are limited (for example, surgery and anesthesiology).

The elasticity of demand facing physician practices. As noted, the elasticity of demand facing individual physicians if they were monopolists would be about -0.2. The elasticity facing perfectly competitive physicians would be negative infinity. The truth must be somewhere between those extremes. There are two methods for estimating this elasticity. These same two methods have been used to estimate the price elasticity of demand facing individual hospitals.

The first uses the information contained in the fact that most physicians are willing to accept below-market prices. For the physician who was just indifferent between accepting assignment on a Medicare case and losing the patient, the marginal cost (including the subjective value of his time) was equal to the Medicare allowance. Taking the average Medicare discount to be 25 percent, we can solve the first-order conditions for a monopolist's profit maximization for the implied elasticity of demand facing the individual physician practice

$$\text{marginal revenue} = \text{marginal cost,}$$

$$= \text{price} \left(1 + \frac{1}{\text{elasticity of demand}}\right) \qquad (4\text{--}1)$$

The resulting price elasticity of demand is -4.0. Physicians who gained by taking assignments either face more elastic demand curves or have lower marginal costs. Those who refused to take assignments either face less elastic demand curves or have higher marginal costs. Probably both are true since those who do not take assignments have been practicing longer and are presumably busier and thus have higher marginal costs. Also, they were of higher quality, at least as measured by such proxies as board certification and the level of their usual fees (Rice and McCall 1983, 52; Rogers and Musacchio 1983, 67). Robert Lee and Jack Hadley (1979) used this approach to estimate the implied elasticities of demand facing physicians of various specialties who make different decisions about accepting assignment. They find implied elasticities ranging from -2.8 to -5.2 for private patients and about -0.4 for the elderly with complete (Medicare and private supplemental) insurance.

The second method is to estimate directly the demand curve facing the physician practices. The literature reports a few of these direct estimates. Using two slightly different ways of modeling insurance coverage, Robert McLean (1980) estimated the firm level demand curves for general practitioners in individual practice as -1.75 and -2.16. He used no measures of quality or amenity. Since higher quality and amenities are correlated with higher prices, this would bias the estimates toward zero. Thus, we can view -1.75 as a lower bound on the average price elasticity facing general practitioners. Unfortunately McLean did not allow the elasticity to vary with insurance coverage, since more complete insurance dramatically reduces the elasticity (Frech and Ginsburg 1975, 1978a, b). Still, this is an important and informative article because it gives one of the few empirical estimates of the firm-level demand elasticities.

Thomas McCarthy (1985) built on McLean's work by adding measures of quality and expanding the set of specialties to include all primary care physicians in fee-for-service practice, such as general and family practitioners, internists, pediatricians, and obstetrician-gynecologists. The data are for 1975, by which time physician insurance was quite common. Quality and amenity are held constant by several measures of waiting time and board certification of the physician. In the demand equation, price is negatively related to physician density but is statistically significant at only the 75–90 percent level. The resulting price elasticities of demand are statistically strong. The estimates vary from -3.07 to -3.32 for different specifications. They are statistically significant at better than the 99.95 percent level, on a one-tailed test (McCarthy 1985, 108–9). These estimates are higher (in absolute value) than those of McLean. This is what one would expect because the omission of quality and amenity biases McLean's estimates downward (toward zero).

Except for the elderly with comprehensive insurance, the estimates from all sources range from -1.75 to -5.2. For primary care physicians, the range of directly estimated elasticities is tighter, from -1.75 to -3.32. While these estimates are far from monopoly, they are all somewhat less elastic than Lester Telser's (1972, chap. 7) estimates of similar price elasticities of demand for individual branded consumer products. There he found price elasticities as high as -17.0. To put these estimates into perspective, let us calculate the percentage markup of price over marginal cost that these elasticities would permit, with the equation above. An elasticity of -1.75 permits a markup of 133 percent over marginal cost, and -3.32 permits a markup of 43 percent, while -5.2 permits a 23 percent markup.

Monopolistic competition. We are left with a picture of the physician services market as monopolistically competitive, with prices constrained by competition but with physicians individually holding market power. This middle-of-the-road view of physician competition suggests that variation in competitiveness across areas and over time is an important element in explaining price variation.[7]

In the application of the theory to physician behavior, a small change in interpretation is necessary. Entry into the profession of medicine is limited. Thus, all physicians earn monopoly rents. There is, however, reasonably free entry across geographical areas and into most specialties. Thus, in equilibrium, the monopoly rent will be equalized across geographic areas and across specialties. The basic analysis is the same, except that the average cost curves include the monopoly rent.

Consumer Information and Competition. The consumer information approach is stressed in the pioneering work of Mark Pauly and Mark Satterthwaite (1981), Joseph Newhouse (1981, 1988) and Mark Satterthwaite (1985). Newhouse argued that more complete insurance depresses incentives to search and reduces the demand elasticities facing individual providers. Thus, he found increasing insurance completeness to be a major explanation for rising hospital prices.

Pauly and Satterthwaite focused on cross-sectional variation in consumer information as a determinant of primary care physician prices. Descriptive sociological studies of consumer choice show that the main source of information is friends and relatives (Lee 1969; Booth

---

7. For monopolistically competitive models applied to physician services markets see Satterthwaite (1985), McGuire (1983), Satterthwaite and Dranove (1991), Hadley (1991), and Pauly (1991).

and Babchuk 1972). Based on this insight, Pauly and Satterthwaite constructed proxies for the costs of consumer information. The percentage of the population that has recently moved and the percentage of families that are female-headed, for example, are negatively related to the size of the consumer's network of associates who recommend doctors. Using 1973 data across large SMSAs, they found prices to be higher where these percentages were higher. The effect they find is the opposite of what Woolley and Frech (1988–1989) found for hospital competition. Pauly and Satterthwaite also examined the effect of increasing the number of physicians in a consumer's market area.

With more physicians in an area, consumer information about each is diluted. It is harder to find more than one acquaintance who has had experience with each individual physician; thus it is harder to track their reputations. Therefore, as the physician density in the market rises, consumer information becomes more costly, and the market power of each individual physician increases. The demand curve facing each physician falls, but it gets steeper. The result is higher prices as physician density in the consumer's market area rises. Pauly and Satterthwaite associated higher densities, not higher citywide physician-to-population ratios, with poorer consumer information. Higher densities were associated with higher prices, while higher physician-to-population ratios were associated with lower ones. Frank Sloan (1982) also found population density to be positively related to fees.

Satterthwaite (1985) presented a formal monopolistic competition model in which higher prices because of more complete insurance or poorer information attracted more physicians. In another formal theoretical model, Thomas McGuire (1983) showed that even superior physicians could gain from reducing consumer information.

At least since Milton Friedman (1962, chap. 9), economists have been saying that group practice in medicine can ease consumers' informational problems. The group develops a reputation for quality and transfers it to individual physicians, much the way a department store does for nonbranded or weakly branded goods. Since the group can outlive an individual, it has excellent incentives to maintain its reputation. This informational benefit of the group should be more valuable in areas where consumer information is poorer. Thomas Getzen (1984) tested this theory by relating the percentage of the population that has moved in the past year to the percentage of physicians practicing in groups across fifty-four large SMSAs in 1975. Population mobility was strongly related to physician membership in groups. If the percentage of households that moved were to rise from 10 to 20 percent, for example, the percentage of the physicians who practiced in groups would rise by 15 percent.

Many of these models depend on higher-quality providers developing a superior reputation that eventually becomes known in the market. Deborah Haas-Wilson (1990) verified this: social workers who received more informed referrals charged higher prices.

The lesson that poorer consumer information translates into more monopoly power for individual providers has not been lost on the providers themselves. As discussed, physicians and other providers have long had "ethical" prohibitions against advertising and other means of informing consumers, which are now being relaxed.

Advertising, price, and quality. Lee Benham (1972) showed that in states that prohibit eyeglass advertising, eyeglasses cost almost twice their price in the least restrictive states. His paper stimulated further research. Following up on the optometry profession, Lee Benham and Alexandra Benham (1975) found that the suppression of consumer information was a key ethical principle of the American Optometric Association. They found that as membership in the association rose from 43 to 91 percent of a state's optometrists, eyeglass prices rose by $12, or 38 percent. In a major Federal Trade Commission study, Ronald Bond and others (1980, 5) found that optometrists in cities allowing advertising charged 24 percent less.

The professions have often argued that advertising and more consumer information would undermine quality. This argument has been carefully studied and decisively rejected for optometry. The FTC study found that quality was about the same on average but varied widely regardless of the advertising rules. This study used an excellent measure of quality: individuals were trained to record their eye examinations, and the results were analyzed by a team of optometrists and scored for thoroughness and accuracy.

John Kwoka (1984) used these data with different econometric tools and a different but highly correlated ($r = 0.71$) measure of quality, the time spent in the eye examination. The mean time for an examination in the restrictive cities was 24 minutes. He found that in cities with advertising, the quality of the advertising optometrists was lower (5 to 21 percent shorter examination), but the quality of the nonadvertising optometrists was higher (50 percent longer examination). The average quality in the advertising cities was higher (21 percent longer examinations), and the average price was lower. Permitting advertising caused average prices to decline by 20 percent, while average quality improved. Other studies of optometry using different data and different models have confirmed these results (Haas-Wilson 1986; Feldman and Begun 1985; Maurizi, Moore, and Shepard 1981). Partly because of this research, the FTC, the courts, and state regulatory authorities have

81

reduced legal and professional obstacles to advertising in the health care fields.

Competition and Medicare's Resource-based Relative Value Scale

Congress has radically changed the way physicians are paid under Medicare. Until 1991, Medicare physician allowances were based on market fees, with adjustments and constraints. By 1996, Medicare physician payment will be based on a nonmarket fee schedule, called the resource-based relative value scale (RBRVS) (Ginsburg, LeRoy, and Hammons 1990; Congressional Budget Office 1990; Physician Payment Review Commission 1990). William Hsiao and the Physician Payment Review Commission constructed the RBRVS, without regard to market fees, from accounting costs and physician time.[8] The new fees will be much lower for surgical procedures (an average reduction of 18 percent) and a bit higher for cognitive medicine. Balance billing will be restricted to 15 percent of the new, lower Medicare allowances.

The RBRVS was first proposed by William Hsiao and William Stason (1979). The idea attracted little attention. One exception was a critical article by Jack Hadley and Robert Berenson (1987). The Department of Health and Human Services rejected the idea and refused to support a large-scale project to construct a workable RBRVS. But Congress favored the RBRVS and forced the DHHS to support the Hsiao project. Since then, the RBRVS has received intensive, and often confidential, review within the government but surprisingly little public debate and analysis. One exception is a conference volume edited by Frech (1991). Unusually little effort has been spent in rationalizing the policy by its proponents (Physician Payment Review Commission 1988, chap. 3; Hsiao and Dunn 1991).

The support for the fee schedule is based on the idea that surgery and related procedures were historically more completely covered by insurance than were office visits, thus competition was weaker in surgery. Therefore, the spread between price and marginal cost is greater for surgery and other procedures than for cognitive medicine. This view implies a large supply of surgeons with light workloads. One small-scale study is supportive (Fuchs 1978), but more research is called for on this topic.

In support of this idea, the RBRVS proponents point out that surgeons' incomes are higher than those of internal medicine and general practice, which are less procedure-oriented. But the monopolistic com-

---

8. For a good general background on the RBRVS and physician market generally, see Frech (1991).

petition model suggests that long-term differences in incomes in different medical specialties must be due to other causes, such as differences in physician ability and artificially limited entry into certain specialties (Satterthwaite and Dranove 1991; Marder and Wilke 1991). Otherwise, entry would equalize the attractiveness (thus roughly the incomes) of the different specialties. We have little understanding of why some specialties earn more than others. Perhaps this lack of understanding should give us a certain amount of caution in adopting a fee schedule whose main purpose is to change the relative fees of different specialties.

Hsiao and Dunn (1991) apparently believe that too much surgery is performed in the United States and that reducing the surgical fees will reduce it. But lower fees imply lower coinsurance, and reduced balance billing also reduces out-of-pocket payment. Thus, the RBRVS will raise demand for surgery among Medicare beneficiaries. Depending on how severe the access (nonprice rationing) of surgery becomes, the volume of surgery may well rise, not fall. Indeed, the Congressional Budget Office (1990) assumes a substantial volume increase in its projections.

Whatever problems might be caused by an inaccurate RBRVS would be both mitigated and illuminated by more-or-less unlimited balance billing. First, the balance billing would eliminate access problems. Any physician would be willing to treat any Medicare patient. Second, the extent of balance billing would show which procedures were mispriced. Underpriced procedures would be balance billed more often and by larger amounts and vice versa. If the system could respond to these market signals, the RBRVS could quickly evolve into a reasonable and efficient system.

Unfortunately, strict limits on balance billing were suggested by the Physician Payment Review Commission (1989) and enacted by Congress in the Omnibus Budget Reconciliation Act of 1989. This limitation will exacerbate the problems caused by inaccuracies in the RBRVS and create mischief itself. The RBRVS will probably cause both access and quality problems for Medicare beneficiaries and possibly higher volume.

5
Supply-induced Demand

Physicians have technical medical knowledge that their customers lack. Thus, consumers demand two different services from physicians: information on health care and the care itself. In the informational role, the physician acts as an agent for the consumer by recommending the health care that he believes is worth its cost to the consumer, considering the out-of-pocket expense, time, risk, and the consumer's preferences and income. This is the case for almost all sellers of services, from lawyers to automobile mechanics, even economic consultants. It is also the case for most goods, especially where their proper choice and use are not self-evident, for example, personal computers. Even for beer and toothpaste and complementary goods and services such as advertising, ease of availability and shelf placement affect sales.

But analysis of the empirical importance of what is called supply-induced demand and how it varies with other economic variables has led to disagreement. Roughly speaking, some economists believe that inducement is empirically important and more common when physician incomes are depressed, either by a greater supply of competing physicians or by regulation. Other economists believe that inducement is not so important empirically and is not systematically related to physician incomes, regulated prices, or the number of competing physicians.

The economists who favor inducement believe that physicians abuse their role as agents. Physicians recommend more medical care than is worthwhile, given its cost and consumers' insurance and medical condition. This can only be considered a type of fraud. Further, the proponents of supply inducement believe that this fraud varies predictably (Evans 1974; Fuchs 1978; Reinhardt 1978, 1985; Dyckman 1978; Rice 1983; Cromwell and Mitchell 1986). That is, as more physicians crowd into a market, they give more fraudulent advice and raise the demand for health care. Thus, more physicians can lead to both more utilization and higher prices. Zachary Dyckman (1978, ii), for example, said that "fees are higher where the relative physician supply is greater. This is consistent with the view that normal market forces are weak or almost nonexistent as constraints on surgical fee inflation."

From these results, some economists would agree with Victor Fuchs (1978, 55): "If the surgeon/population ratio should increase . . . the result will probably be higher rather than lower fees, and also more operations."

Inducement Theory

Robert Evans (1974) has presented a theoretical argument, based on a utility-maximizing model of the physician. This model and variants have been thoroughly analyzed by Frank Sloan and Roger Feldman (1978), Ewe Reinhardt (1978), and James Ramsey (1980).[1] These writers have concluded that there are few differences between the standard or neoclassical model and the inducement model in comparative statics, thus in predictions of relations among variables. The so-called standard model simply rules out all systematic variation in inducement.[2] Further, the inducement model is difficult either to refute or confirm with ordinary market data. Positive or negative correlations of a physician-to-population ratio with quantity or fees, for example, are consistent with it.

Can More Physicians Lead to Higher Fees? A major piece of evidence supporting the inducement model is the observation that the physician-to-population ratio is sometimes positively correlated with fees. Given that the physician-to-population ratio is exogenous or an exogenous instrument for it can be found, this contradicts the so-called standard model in which an increase in supply causes the equilibrium price–quantity combination to move down the demand curve and result in lower fees.

In the inducement model, there are offsetting effects. The usual effect of moving down the demand curve remains. In addition, more competing physicians leads to lower incomes and fewer busy physicians—and more inducement. Some (for example, Dyckman 1978) believe that the inducement may move the demand curve out far enough

---

1. David Dranove (1988) has presented a theoretical model of inducement where there is no ethical value or constraint. The only ill effect of inducement is damage to the physician's reputation. This reduces his future income. As a result, it can be profitable for physicians to collude to give honest advice (not induce).

2. The terminology used in this literature is misleading at best. From a theoretical viewpoint, the inducement model is not at all unorthodox. It is a minor generalization of the so-called standard model, allowing for nonprice competition and advertising. Such models have been used for decades by such economists as Peter Steiner, George Stigler, Lester Telser, and Michael Spence.

to offset the increased supply and lead to higher output per physician and higher fees.

A large movement in the demand curve is necessary for fees to rise because of more physicians in the area. The demand curve facing the individual physician must expand beyond its original position and raise both his output and fees. For fees to rise while output per physician falls would require the elasticity of demand facing each individual physician to fall. Nothing in the inducement model or literature suggests this demand-side change.

The physician's relative distaste for inducement must be extremely sensitive to his level of utility for fees to rise from an exogenous increase in the physician-to-population ratio. His utility function must be strongly nonhomothetic.[3] In the new equilibrium, the physician is earning more than before the introduction of additional competing physicians but inducing more. At his new optimum, he has a lower level of utility, with higher earnings, more work, and more inducement: financial earnings and wealth are inferior goods, and reducing inducement is a strongly superior good. A slight reduction in the attainable combinations of financial wealth and inducement leads to such a large increase in inducement that financial income rises. This theory gives strong predictions for the physician's response to changes in his individual demand curve (Sloan and Feldman 1978).

If more complete insurance becomes commonplace, for example, the physician will choose to induce less and have lower earnings, supply fewer services and charge less. This prediction is routinely falsified (Sloan and Feldman 1978, 51; Reinhardt 1978, 135). Thus, the requirements for the inducement model to be consistent with an increase in physician-to-population ratio causing an increase in fees are improbable.

Competition and Inducement. Some economists believe that physician inducement makes procompetitive policies less attractive. Yet, another approach to modeling inducement, attributed to Miron Stano (1987), argues that their concern is misplaced. Stano analogized inducement to advertising in the standard profit-maximizing model of firm behavior (Dorfman and Steiner 1954). Inducement costs the physician resources, but it raises demand. Thus, inducement leads to greater

---

3. Nonhomothetic utility functions imply that the individual's relative valuation of goods and bads varies as his level of utility or income rises. Here a small decrease in utility resulting from a small decrease in demand facing each physician must make him much more willing to give distasteful fraudulent advice to his patients.

profits, up to a point. At the optimum, the firm equates the marginal cost of additional inducement per unit of sales to the profit it gets on that additional unit. The higher the profit, the greater the incentive to induce demand.

Thus, the amount of inducement depends on the markup of price over marginal cost, which itself depends on the degree of monopoly power of the physician. The more monopoly power, the greater the markup and the more inducement. Policies that make the market more competitive, thus reduce the markup of price over marginal cost, reduce the incentive for inducement.[4] In the extreme, if the market were

---

4. At the optimum of the profit-maximizing monopoly we know that the elasticity of demand, price, and marginal cost are related by

$$\frac{p}{p-c} = -\eta, \tag{5-1}$$

where

p = price,
c = marginal cost,
η = price elasticity of demand.
Turning to the inducement, the physician's quantity sold depends on price and inducement:

$$q = q(p, i), \tag{5-2}$$

where

q = quantity,
i = inducement, measured in dollars.
Profit is then

$$\pi = pq - cq - i. \tag{5-3}$$

At a profit maximum, the marginal profit of inducement is equal to zero (assuming decreasing returns to inducement so that second-order conditions are met):

$$\frac{\partial \pi}{\partial i} = p \cdot \frac{\partial q}{\partial i} - c \cdot \frac{\partial q}{\partial i} - 1 = 0. \tag{5-4}$$

Rearranging, we get

$$\frac{p}{p-c} = p \cdot \frac{\partial q}{\partial i}. \tag{5-5}$$

The right hand side is just the marginal value product of inducement ($MVP(i)$, and the left-hand side is the negative of the price elasticity of demand. Therefore

$$-\eta = MVP(i). \tag{5-6}$$

At the optimum, the marginal value product of inducement is equated to to become perfectly competitive, there would be no monopoly markup and no inducement. Following Stano's view, it seems highly likely that more competition would decrease inducement.

One's attitude toward competition and inducement are not logically linked. Economists who strongly believe in inducement might favor competition to reduce it. Or if they have a slightly different picture of how inducement works, they might believe that competition would make matters worse.

Alternative Theories

Several other theories can explain the stylized facts of a positive correlation between the physician-to-population ratio and prices or utilization.

Increasing Monopoly in Monopolistic Competition. The model of Pauly and Satterthwaite (1981), discussed above, is an example of an alternative theory. Based on the theory of monopolistic competition, they argued that more physicians in the market degrade consumers' information about each physician.[5] This process decreases the elasticity of demand facing individual physicians and allows them to raise prices. The higher prices attract more physicians to the area.

Satterthwaite (1985) developed the monopolistic competition theory more formally. He said that, whatever the cause, poorer consumer information leads to less elastic demand, thus higher prices. The higher prices attract more physicians and lead to a higher physician-to-population ratio. In monopolistically competitive equilibrium, demand curves are tangent to cost curves. In areas with less elastic demand curves facing individual physician firms, the tangency must occur at

---

minus the price elasticity of demand facing the individual physician. As the market becomes more competitive, that value rises (the elasticity itself gets more negative). Since there are diminishing returns to inducement, this situation requires less inducement in more competitive environments, where price is closer to marginal costs.

5. The usual model of monopolistic competition assumes free entry. In the application of the theory to physician behavior, a small change in interpretation is necessary. Entry into the profession of medicine is limited. Thus, all physicians can earn monopoly rents in a monopolistically competitive equilibrium. Among physicians, however, there is reasonably free entry across geographic areas and into most specialties. Thus, in equilibrium, the monopoly rent will be equalized across geographic areas and across specialties. The basic analysis is the same except that the average cost curves that are tangent to the demand curves include the monopoly rent.

lower levels of output per physician and higher prices. These areas of higher prices must have more physicians.

A major causes of poorer information is more complete insurance. High-price, physician-rich areas are likely to have more demand per capita, thus higher utilization. These areas are also likely to contain more specialized physicians and more sophisticated hospitals and cater to a larger geographical area and treat more exotic ailments.

Time Costs. Arthur De Vany, Donald House, and Thomas Saving (1983) argued that where providers are more numerous, patient time costs are lower. This increase in quality raises demand and money price (but not total price, which is the sum of money and time prices). The positive relation between provider-population ratio and low time cost leads to a positive relation of providers to money fees.

Tryfon Beazoglou, Dennis Heffley, and Subhash Ray (1986) presented a variant of that model, concentrating on spatial analysis and travel time. Entry leads to lower travel time and lower total price, but the money price can rise. Physicians are assumed to interact strategically as if they were perfectly colluding.[6] The authors showed that entry, which leads to smaller market areas per physician, reduces the total price for the average consumer and moves into a less elastic region of his demand curve. By reducing the money price elasticity of demand, entry can cause higher money prices. Therefore, areas with more physicians can have higher money prices but require less consumer time and thus have lower total prices. The authors reported that experimentation with lower conjectural variations, consistent with more competition, can reverse the result that money price rises with entry.

Excess Demand and Nonprice Rationing. For markets with excess demand, there is a simple and convincing alternative to the inducement theory. An early version was sketched by William Comanor (1980, 4–21). In this situation, the providers must engage in nonprice rationing. One would hope that the care would be rationed, at least partly, based on medical factors. But even technically perfectly professional rationing is economically imperfect and inefficient. Physicians have no information or incentive to ration in accord with consumer preferences regarding risk and other factors.

A common form of nonprice rationing, for example, is to stop taking new patients. Price controls and excess demand also eliminate the

---

6. Formally, the authors assume a conjectural variation of 1.0. That means that each seller responds to the increase in output of his rivals by matching it.

incentive to practice in less pleasant inner cities and rural areas. The same lack of incentives would affect specialty choice and the general style of practice.

Price controls under national health insurance have caused physician migration away from rural areas in developed countries (Frech and Ginsburg 1978b, 37–41). Researchers found that when Quebec instituted universal health insurance, the style of practice changed to favor the physicians' preferences, not the consumers' preferences. Home visits dropped by 63 percent; office visits rose by 32 percent. Physician time per office visit declined by 16 percent. Also, doctors' hours of work per day dropped from 10.3 to 8.8. Simultaneously physicians' real net incomes rose 35 percent in two years (Comanor 1980, 16–18; Enterline 1973, 1975).

More important for our purposes, excess demand and nonprice rationing lead to an empirical correlation between the physician-to-population ratio and utilization, even in the absence of inducement. When there is excess demand, there is no need for inducement. Consumers demand more care than providers are willing to supply. Physicians can supply as much as they like, without ever abusing the agency relationship. For various reasons, some areas will be physician-rich. Therefore, utilization per person will be higher in physician-rich areas.

This theory applies directly to areas where price controls are binding. This analysis applies to Americans with Medicaid insurance and national health insurance plans with price-controlled fee-for-service medical care. It also includes the members of some private or semiprivate health insurance plans where fee-for-service physicians are not allowed to balance bill. The sickness funds of Germany and Switzerland are good examples. Although the situation is less clear, it probably also applies to medically underserved areas in the United States even in the absence of explicit price control.

For subtle reasons of professional, governmental, or insurance pressure, fees do not seem to rise enough in such areas to clear the market. Even in the United States, at least for some specialties, physicians engage in nonprice rationing. The addition of more physicians softens the nonprice rationing and therefore raises utilization. The additional physicians do not put downward pressure on prices until there are enough of them to clear the market and end the excess demand.

It is also interesting to consider the introduction of, or increase in, consumer copayments in markets with excess demand. One would expect little change in total utilization until the increased copayments reduce demand enough to clear the market. The level of copayment necessary for market clearing will differ among physicians. Typically some physicians in particular areas, or specialties, or perhaps new to the market, do not face excess demand. Even small changes in copayment would affect their utilization.

Even if total utilization were little changed, additional coinsurance in a national health insurance system might be good public policy. It would reduce the magnitude of the excess demand gap and increase the influence of consumers' preferences and values on the mixture and style of practice. Thus, the actual mixture of service provided would reflect true consumer preferences and values more and physician preferences less. Even if the higher coinsurance did not reduce costs, it would make the system both more efficient and more humane in that it would respond more to consumers' values.

Empirical Research

There has been much research on physician fees and quantities, much of it surveyed by Sloan and Feldman (1978) and by Feldman and Sloan (1988). In many, but not all, of the cross-sectional studies, the physician-to-population ratio has been positively associated with fees. This association has often been interpreted as rejecting the standard model and proving that inducement is important. But another, simpler hypothesis appears to make more sense.

Physician Location and the Identification Problem. As Richard Auster and Ronald Oaxaca (1981) showed, it is difficult statistically to identify supplier-induced demand. I suspect that the empirical results reflect physician locational decisions, not inducement. More physicians are attracted to areas with more demand for their services. These areas will have higher utilization and physician-to-population ratios. This case, and the other theories discussed above, can explain the positive correlation of the physician-to-population ratio to utilization without recourse to demand-inducement theories.

The extent of physician competition varies across market areas, mostly because of variations in consumer information and insurance. In less competitive areas, the demand curves facing the individual physicians will be less elastic, so the profit or utility maximizing price will be higher. In equilibrium, physicians can obtain the same level of utility or income everywhere; where the price is high, utilization per physician would have to be low. Cross-sectional econometrics typically compares long-run equilibriums.

The importance of physician migration is reinforced by the finding that physicians are mobile and responsive to income opportunities (Newhouse, Williams, Bennett, and Schwartz 1982; Benham, Maurizi, and Reder 1968). Therefore, these cross-sectional analyses are contaminated by simultaneous equations bias. Also, Newhouse and others show that as their numbers have increased over time, specialists have located in progressively smaller and smaller cities. Inducement cannot be easy and effective, or the specialists would have stayed in the favored large cities and simply induced demand to raise their incomes.

Some analysts have tried to account for the bias problem of simultaneous equations by using two-stage least squares. A notable example is the work on state data of Victor Fuchs and Marcia Kramer (1972). The technique requires exogenous variables that strongly affect the physician-to-population ratio but are unrelated to demand. Unfortunately, the variables used in this analysis to identify an exogenous increase in the physician-to-population ratio are typical economic and health care variables, which are not exogenous with respect to demand.

Waiting Time and Quality. The quality of services is likely to be higher where there are more physicians. Travel and waiting time, for example, would be lower. This higher quality would raise demand. Both travel and waiting time have been found—by Jan Acton (1975), Thomas McCarthy (1985), and Marilyn Manser and Elizabeth Fineman (1983)—to affect the demand for physician care. Travel and waiting time appear even more important for dentistry, according to Arthur De Vany, Donald House, and Thomas Saving (1983). Controlling for waiting time reverses the positive correlation of dental fees with the dentist-population ratio (De Vany, House, and Saving 1983, 679).[7]

Waiting time can be subtle and difficult to measure. If doctors require patients to return for several visits unnecessarily, for example, there is no obvious waiting. But consumer time is wasted, and this waste reduces demand; thus it helps clear the market (Danzon 1993).

Quality aspects other than waiting time are generally ignored for lack of data. The omission of waiting time is less serious for surgery; hence some research has focused on that specialty. Some argue that because insurance coverage has typically been better for surgery, inducement behavior is more likely for surgery. Consistent with this argument is the finding in one small-scale study that surgeons were significantly less busy than other specialists (Hughes, Fuchs, Jacoby, and Lewit 1972). But this interesting study has not been replicated.

---

7. Consumer waiting time also allows for better use of the physician's time. Thus, longer consumer waiting time in the office leads to higher output (Headen 1991).

Surgery. Focusing on surgeons and using urban area (SMSA) data for 1963 and 1970, Victor Fuchs (1978) introduced an interesting innovation. He used the per capita hotel and motel receipts of the area to try to identify the supply of physicians. The receipts are a proxy for the nonpecuniary attractiveness of the area to physicians but are arguably exogenous with respect to health care demand. Areas with high hotel expenditures are likely to have more physicians per capita than others. This variable is probably the least contaminated with economic or demand influences. But Charles Phelps (1986, 363) pointed out that any local area that is attractive to mobile physicians is also attractive to high-income, mobile, retired people. Even this variable is confounded with demand variation.

In related work of my own, using 1970 SMSA data, the addition of the hotel variable to a regression containing several conventional economic variables added nothing to the explanation of physician-to-population ratios. Clearly the hotel variable could not be used to identify exogenous variation in the physician-to-population ratio in that data.

Fuchs found that higher surgeon-population ratios were associated with higher fees and utilization. The Fuchs study of surgeons has been extended with a superior and larger data set of pooled time-series (1969 to 1976), cross-sectional data by Jerry Cromwell and Janet Mitchell (1986). Following Fuchs, no quality measures are included. In an attempt to expand on Fuchs's hotel receipts variable, urbanization, the presence of colleges, racial mix, and climate (measured as temperature) are added. Urbanization and racial mix are clearly demand variables. Climate is mismeasured since weather can be too hot as well as too cold. (Perhaps the Boston location of the researchers led them to forget this point.) And the hotel variable, the only possibly legitimate one, is not powerful enough. Therefore, two-stage least squares will not identify the effect of exogenous variation in the surgeon-population ratio.

The results with the whole sample are similar to Fuchs's 1978 analysis. Higher surgeon-population ratios are associated with higher surgery rates and especially with higher prices for surgery. The estimated elasticity of price with respect to the surgeon-population ratio is close to unity, 0.9. This is about twice the estimate that Fuchs (1978, 135, 145) obtained. Cromwell and Mitchell interpret this as evidence for inducement. This study was done about as well as possible, given the data limitations, but there are many problems of measurement and specification errors, discussed by Phelps (1986). Insurance completeness is measured poorly. The specification and measurement problems, plus the lack of identification of an exogenous supply variation, undermine their claim of having discovered and measured an inducement effect.

Subsamples. Cromwell and Mitchell went on to estimate their equations on subsamples. The estimates shed considerable light on physician pricing, even if they are not decisive on the inducement hypothesis.

City size. First, Cromwell and Mitchell split the sample into nonmetropolitan areas, small SMSAs (less than 500,000 population), and large SMSAs. The results differ enormously. In the nonmetropolitan areas, higher surgeon-population ratios are not associated with more utilization. Further, more surgeons reduce prices, with an elasticity of about −0.2. In large SMSAs, the results are similar to the full sample except that the elasticity of price with respect to the surgeon-population ratio is only about 0.7, less than the full sample. The small SMSAs fall about halfway between, with the elasticity of price about 0.5.

This variation across subsamples implies that the aggregation of the full sample might be misleading. More important, the variance supports the idea that consumer information is poorer in large cities and worsens as the number of physicians increases (Pauly and Satterthwaite 1981; Satterthwaite 1985). Cromwell and Mitchell also tried to test the Pauly and Satterthwaite model directly by entering the number of surgeons per square mile into the regression. Surprisingly, and in conflict with other studies, it had no effect (1986, 307). Clearly, more analysis of this effect of physician density would be useful.

Mark Pauly (1980b, 82–90) also analyzed subsamples. Instead of surgery, he used office visits as the dependent variable. He did not try to identify the exogenous effect of physician-to-population ratio. He simply used ordinary least squares. The observations were of individual families, with the data taken from a large survey.[8] Pauly found little availability effect when estimating the total sample. He disaggregated the data by size of city and according to the education level of the head of the household. The latter is a proxy for the consumer's general level of information. He found no effect of physician-to-population ratio in small cities, regardless of the education level of the consumer, consistent with Cromwell and Mitchell. Pauly found a small but statistically

---

8. The use of micro (individual) data may disguise the simultaneous equations problem, but it does not eliminate it. The data still arise from a market where physician location is a result of economic forces—representing a supply curve of physicians to a particular area.

significant effect for the lesser-educated consumers in large cities and a large but negative effect for the better-educated consumers in large cities. Pauly concluded that the inducement effect was small.

Surgeon "shortage" and "surplus" areas. In an attempt to test whether excess demand is the cause of the positive association of more surgeons with more utilization, Cromwell and Mitchell split the sample according to surgeon workload. They split the sample at the mean value of 280 operations per year into "surplus" (low surgeon workload) or "shortage" (high surgeon workload) areas. Again, the results in the subsamples differed.

In shortage areas, demand variables were not important—as one would expect if there were nonprice rationing and excess demand. The surgeon-population ratio explains much of the variation in utilization. The elasticity of utilization with respect to the ratio is 0.28, far higher than the 0.09 in the full sample. In the surplus area, conversely, demand variables are important, more so than in the full sample. The effect of the surgeon-population ratio on utilization is far less, with an elasticity of 0.08.

Even if this elasticity were measuring the inducement effect, the effect is weakest in areas with an abundance of surgeons, the areas where there is a policy concern with it. Also, the results show that some, perhaps most, of the observed correlations used to argue for inducement are due to excess demand. This brings us to the next type of empirical study.

Insured Populations under Price Control. There have been several attempts to test for the presence of supplier-induced demand for populations under price control. Since the prices are regulated and more or less uniform in these systems, the attention of researchers turns to the relation of the physician-to-population ratio and utilization or costs.

Canada. Philip Held and Larry Manheim (1980) examined the effect of the physician-to-population ratio, treated as exogenous, on the costs of treatment for hypertension among a sample of about 13,000 Quebec residents. The study covers the first five years of Quebec's 100 percent coverage health insurance plan. In their preferred specification of the regression, Held and Manheim found a statistically significant elasticity of costs with respect to the general practitioner–to–population ratio of about 0.12. The specialist-to-population ratio had, surprisingly, a negative effect about one fourth as large.

Using utilization in eight payment districts over the three fiscal years 1972–1975, William Comanor (1980) performed a similar analysis for Ontario. He presented both ordinary least-squares and two-stage least-squares results. The results are similar. But the general practitioner- and specialist-to-population ratios are identified only with traditional medical and economic variables; thus, the coefficients are biased upward. This work is interesting because of the different effects of different types of physicians. The elasticity of utilization with respect to specialists per capita is high, 0.93. The elasticity for general practitioners is negative, −0.22. Apparently, when specialists take over patients from general practitioners, they spend far more. The combined elasticity for increasing both types of physicians proportionally is 0.71 (1980, 30). Comanor was careful to note that these results cannot distinguish among the three competing explanations: demand inducement, excess demand, and savings in time costs (1980, 22–23).

Switzerland. Kornelius Kraft and Matthias von der Schulenberg (1986) found similar results for data from individual physicians in the Swiss canton of Berne. Twenty-eight areas were used to measure the physician-to-population ratios. Since the canton itself is small, these areas are likewise small; on the average, they contain only thirty-two physicians. The patients are all members of Swiss sickness funds, which negotiate total prices and do not allow balance billing, much like the Quebec health insurance scheme. But the Swiss funds require a 10 percent coinsurance, while there is no coinsurance in Quebec.

Kraft and Schulenberg reported an elasticity of cost per patient with respect to the physician-to-population ratio of about 0.37. With such small areas, one might suspect much border crossing, which would confuse the results. But the authors found that whether the data are defined by the location of the patients or the doctors, the results are similar. They attempted to treat the physician-to-population ratio endogenously and identified it by the number of hospital beds in the local area. Because this variable is confounded with demand for convenience of the patients if no other reason, the exogenous effect of the physician-to-population ratio has not been found. Kraft and Schulenberg found almost the same results whether the physician-to-population ratio was treated as exogenous, with ordinary least squares, or was treated as endogenous, with two-stage least-squares (1986, 374).

They then applied the Hausman test of the endogeneity of the physician-to-population ratio. This test, in effect, compares the ordinary least-squares estimates (perhaps tainted by simultaneous equation bias) with those of the two-stage least-squares estimates (assumed unbiased but possibly inefficient) to see if they are significantly different. Not surprisingly, the test fails to reject the hypothesis that the estimates are identical. Under the assumption that the two-stage estimates are identified and free of bias themselves, Kraft and Schulenberg concluded that the physician-to-population ratio is exogenous.

It seems more likely that the two-stage estimate is contaminated with demand influences (Nelson and Startz 1990). Both estimates are overstated almost equally by simultaneous equations bias, and one cannot conclude anything about the degree of exogeneity of the physician-to-population ratio.

In a later study using Swiss and German data, von der Schulenberg (1989) finds both higher physician/population ratios and higher utilization in urban areas, as compared with rural areas. He attributes both results to lower time costs for both waiting and travel in these areas.

These studies overstate the effect of exogenous physician-to-population ratios on utilization. But undoubtedly if someone could identify the exogenous effect, it would be positive and probably large enough to be economically important. Nevertheless, the effect cannot necessarily be attributed to inducement. Nonprice rationing in a situation of excess demand is more likely the main explanation.

Medicare and price control. It has been observed that when Medicare fees or allowances are reduced, utilization rises and defeats the cost-containment goal of the price controls. Thomas Rice (1983) found this for a natural experiment in Colorado where Medicare allowances were cut in urban areas. Jack Hadley and Robert Lee (1978–1979) reported the same increase in utilization under the Nixon price controls of 1972–1974. Under the controls, utilization rose so rapidly that total expenditures rose faster under price control than when the controls were released in 1975. And the Congressional Budget Office (1986, 7) found a similar increase in utilization during the Medicare fee freeze (price controls) that began July 1, 1984. Physician services expenditures in constant dollars rose by 10.8 percent during 1985, the first full year of the fee freeze. During 1984, only half of which experienced the fee freeze, expenditures rose by only 2.1 percent. Although most authors do not take a position on inducement, Rice (1983) did. He interpreted the perverse effect of price controls as inducement to offset a cut in fees (1983).

There is, however, a simple alternative explanation. The price controls caused a large reduction in the out-of-pocket payments paid by Medicare beneficiaries. This was especially true of those who were paying balance bills. Over the first year and one-half, the 1984 freeze, the consumer price index rose by 5.6 percent. Based on inflation rates, physician fees would have risen by 1.5 percent more, or 7.1 percent. By the end of the period, inflation-adjusted physician prices were 7.1 percent lower than they would have been in the absence of the freeze. For beneficiaries whose physicians did not change their decision about accepting assignment and whose Medigap insurance, if any, paid proportionally, this would have reduced their out-of-pocket payments by 7.1 percent. Given an elasticity of demand of about −0.2, utilization for this group would have risen by 1.5 percent more than it would have without the freeze.

Perhaps even more important, the freeze included many inducements for physicians to accept assignment and therefore not balance bill. These inducements were successful. The assignment rate, after nine years of stability between 50.5 and 54.0 percent, rose abruptly from 53.9 percent in 1983 to 59.0 percent in 1984 to 68.5 percent in 1985 (Congressional Budget Office 1986, 23). The switch to accepting assignment led to a large decrease in out-of-pocket price, more than 50 percent for beneficiaries without Medigap insurance. For beneficiaries with Medigap insurance that covered the coinsurance but not the balance bill, the switch to accepting assignment caused a 100 percent drop in out-of-pocket price. One would expect large increases in utilization of doctors who started accepting assignments in 1985.

Physician-initiated Visits and the Physician as Agent. In the face of doubt that the traditional studies could detect induced demand, Louis Rossiter and Gail Wilensky (1981) tried a novel approach with data from the large National Medical Care Expenditure Survey, which distinguished whether the physician or the consumer initiated the visit. Of the total visits, 36 percent were initiated by physicians. The authors calculated the physician-initiated expenditures for both ambulatory care and for all care (including all inpatient hospital care). They related these variables to many demand variables and to local surgeon- and physician-to-population ratios, presumably measured at the county level.

The results give a unique picture of how the physician functions as agent of the consumer. We would expect (and hope) that physicians would initiate more expenditures for patients in poorer health or with more complete insurance or with higher income. Especially for regions and populations where excess demand is important, we would expect a higher physician-to-population ratio to raise expenditures, even without inducement. Exogenous variation in the physician-to-population ratio is no better identified here than in other studies. Nonetheless, this study gives us the best picture yet of the agency relationship.

The results are fascinating. Physician-initiated care is found to be sensitive to the level of insurance whether it is measured by dummies for different types or by an estimate of net price. The elasticity of physician-initiated ambulatory care with respect to net price was 0.57. When the dummies were used, there were large effects. Consumers with Medicare plus private Medigap insurance, for example, incurred $289, or 50 percent more, in total expenses and $60 or 40 percent more physician-initiated ambulatory expenses than those with Medicare only. The health status measures also had large effects, as did age. The elasticity of physician-initiated ambulatory care with respect to the percent of visits with chronic conditions was 0.137. The elasticity with respect to age ranged from 0.421 to 0.448. The percentage of physicians who were board certified was strongly negative to total expenditures (elasticity at means of −0.112) and positive to ambulatory expenditures (elasticity of 0.059). Both estimates were significant at the 90 percent level. The mean percentage board certified was 55.9.

The effects of variation in physician abundance were small. In the total expenditures regressions, the surgeon-population ratio had almost no effect, with an elasticity of 0.006 and a t-statistic of only 0.55 (in a sample of 18,442). In considering the remaining simultaneous equations bias and the likelihood of excess demand in some places for some groups, this finding is consistent with no effect at all. There was a measurable effect on physician-initiated ambulatory care, with an elasticity of 0.074 or 0.106, depending on the treatment of insurance coverage in the equation.[9] Again, in considering the simultaneous equations bias and the possibility of excess demand for some populations in some areas, this is a small effect indeed. From this analysis, the authors concluded that "the initiation of expenditures by physicians appears to be dominated by factors consistent with the physician's role as agent rather than by factors that reflect only self-interest" (Rossiter and Wilensky 1984, 242).

Additional insight into the physician's agency relationship has been provided by studies of consumer information. Better informed consumers would be less prey to inducement since inducement is based on misleading consumers about what medical care is actually in their own interest.

John Bunker and Byron Brown (1974) focused on surgery, which is believed to be more prone to inducement than other specialties. To test this proposition, Bunker and Brown compared surgery rates for physicians and their spouses with those of other professionals. The results were striking: the physicians and their spouses consumed more surgery than the other professionals.

In a similar vein, Donald Kenkel (1990) related objectively measured health knowledge to health care utilization. Consistent with

---

9. Inexplicably, the authors give slightly different elasticities, 0.11 to 0.13, in the text (Rossiter and Wilensky 1984, 241).

Bunker and Brown, he found that better informed consumers used more medical care. Even though highly insured, the consumers used less medical care than the physicians thought appropriate. This suggests that, *ceteris paribus*, a more professionally dominated system would raise costs, not reduce them.

Consumer Information. As discussed, Pauly and Satterthwaite (1981) examined a model of physician pricing across the one hundred largest cities. They found a positive relationship between the physician-to-population ratio and fees using traditional specifications. But when they held constant several measures of consumer information, the effect of more physicians in the city on prices became negative, while the effect of more physicians in the consumers' immediate market area remained positive. They concluded that the presence of more physicians, at least in large cities, made consumer information worse and by that token raised prices. While they have clearly shown that consumer information is important for physician pricing, the argument that more physicians, in itself, hinders information is more controversial.

Time Series versus Cross-Section. It appears impossible to identify the exogenous impact of changes in the physician-to-population ratio in cross-sectional analysis. These studies are subject to a bias in the direction of falsely showing a positive effect of more physicians on both use and price. In contrast, much of the variation in physician-to-population ratio over time has been due to political pressures largely unrelated to the demand and supply for physician services. Thus, in time series, the physician-to-population ratio can be taken as exogenous.

Early analysis ran into econometric problems, as critiqued in Newhouse, Phelps, and Marquis (1980). More recent work has been more successful. Hall and Lindsay (1980), Leffler and Lindsay (1981), and Noether (1986) found that the aggregate U.S. physician-to-population ratio has a strong negative relationship to physician incomes. Similar results have been found in Canada. Since cross-sectional analyses often find weakly negative relationships, these studies are only suggestive.

Fortunately, one time series study by Jesse Hixon and Nina Mocniak (1980) focused on the price of physician and dental services. They found normal supply-and-demand functions and a strong price-depressing effect from increasing the number of physicians and dentists. This is strong evidence that supplier-induced demand is not powerful enough to raise prices as the number of providers rises exogenously. The positive correlation of physician-to-population ratio to fees that is sometimes seen in cross-section studies apparently reflects simultaneous equations bias, not inducement.

In summary, despite all the attention paid to the supply-induced demand idea, it does not seem to be a major factor in physician market behavior. Data cited as evidence generally can be explained quite satisfactorily in other ways. Data that allow more definitive interpretation show small effects. Thus, economic and policy analysis can proceed with concepts of monopolistically competitive markets that are simpler and clearer.

6
Competition among Health Insurers

All health insurers, broadly defined, either provide medical care or contract to pay medical bills in return for a fixed premium. This contract provides the service of risk pooling or risk transferring. The insurer, or sometimes the employer for large groups, takes the risk of incurring high medical bills in return for the premium. The cost of this service can be broken down into two parts: (1) the expected loss or expected benefit payment and (2) the loading charge, the difference between the expected loss and the premium. The loading charge covers the insurer's administrative costs, risk premium, and profits. Competition among insurers affects the size of the loading charge.

From a social or public policy viewpoint, the size of the loading charge is the least important and least controversial aspect of health insurance. Most important, insurance has profound effects on the level of expenditures for health care.

American health insurance is undergoing extensive change. Traditional insurance, from both Blue Cross/Blue Shield and from the commercial insurers, was essentially a subsidy of health care, with little control of the resulting increased utilization and price. This type of insurance is rapidly disappearing. In its place, the insurer is involved in both the price and quantity decisions in health care utilization in the form of PPOs, HMOs, and other managed-care organizations. Although employer "self-insurance" is becoming more common, this new form hardly affects the analysis of most issues.

Insurance and Health Care Interactions

Health insurance influences health care in many ways. It raises demand, reduces competition among providers, and encourages technological innovation to proceed in certain directions.

Moral Hazard. First, and best understood of the interactions, is the concept of moral hazard. In a classic (1968) article, Mark Pauly brought the idea from the insurance industry into general use in economics. Moral hazard results from insurance reducing the out-of-pocket price of health care at the time of purchase. This process leads consumers to purchase more care than they would have without insurance. The type of care demanded is also changed by the subsidy of health insurance. The health care is more costly (more intense, higher quality, and more convenient) as well. To some extent, this change in demand is an efficient and rational response to a higher wealth level where one is sick. But most of the increase in demand is wasteful.

Optimal use of health care. We need a benchmark for optimal health care use. The type of insurance contract that would lead to this optimal use is unobtainable in the real world, but its analysis illuminates the problem of moral hazard. Optimal use of health care would occur if consumers had insurance that transferred wealth or income across states of the world (that is, sick versus not sick) but did not distort prices. That is, the insurance would provide a lump-sum payment if the consumer were to become ill, but the consumer could spend the additional wealth any way he saw fit. If he purchased health care with it, he would still pay the full market price for it. Therefore, all health care purchased would be worth its full value to the consumer. This type of insurance is called a contingent claim or an Arrow-Debreu claim. While contingent claim insurance is impossible for most health care coverage, it is closely approximated for other types of insurance.

Auto collision insurance, for example, pays a lump sum, depending on estimates of the extent of the damage. Usually the consumer can repair the car to a greater or lesser extent than the amount of the insurance payment. Thus, there is no moral hazard induced in the auto repair business by the insurance. Similarly, fire insurance pays a lump sum in the event of damage, and the consumer decides what to do with the payment. Ordinarily, the policyholder is given the choice of whether to build the same size house, a larger house, a small house, or nothing at all.[1]

In residential fire insurance, the demand for repair services is raised somewhat simply because the consumer is wealthier in the bad state of the world (a fire). Thus, there is a wealth effect specific to that state of the world that raises the demand for home repair services. But these state-specific wealth effects are not inefficient. Consumers still face the true prices for purchasing repair services. Given their higher

---

1. Homeowner's insurance paying replacement cost is different. To get the higher payment, one must actually rebuild the house in the same configuration as the original. To vary the plan requires negotiation with the insurer.

wealth, they purchase the optimal amount of them. Even though insurance raises demand for repairs, this is not moral hazard.

An appealing benchmark for the correct amount of health care is the amount that an informed consumer with this hypothetical contingent claim insurance would purchase. Actual health insurance unfortunately is far from this ideal. Since there is usually no reasonably objective way to determine just what the damage to a person is as a result of an illness or accident, there is no basis for a lump-sum contingent payment. Instead, insurance simply subsidizes medical care by paying a varying proportion of the bill. As a result of the subsidy, the consumer demands care beyond the amount where it is worth its cost.

Moral hazard leads to a loss of consumer welfare equal to the difference between the cost of production of the excessive units of health care and their value to the consumer. Thus, we can speak of different types of insurance leading to more or less welfare loss. Clearly the worst moral hazard losses would come from insurance that paid 100 percent of medical bills and exercised no controls on utilization.[2]

Consumer copayment. Moral hazard losses can be reduced by decreasing the extent of the subsidy. In practice, this is accomplished largely by requiring that the consumer pay deductibles, coinsurance, or balance bills in excess of an allowed benefit level per unit service. This is a powerful and reliable method of reducing costs. But higher copayments increase the financial risk facing the consumer. Setting the optimal out-of-pocket payment requires balancing higher financial risk with more efficient health care consumption.

Managed care. Another approach is for the insurer to impose non-price controls on the consumer's utilization.[3] Many methods can accomplish this. The most prominent is the HMO, in which the insurer and the provider are combined. The insurer is paid a fixed premium amount per capita (called capitation) and agrees to provide whatever health care is needed. The insurer-provider has the short-run incentive

---

2. Some early discussion focused the blame for overuse and high cost of hospital care on cost-based reimbursement, which was traditionally used by a majority of Blue Cross plans. (The other plans paid hospital charges.) But Mark Pauly and David Drake (1970) showed convincingly that the real culprit was overly complete insurance; the form of reimbursement had no effect. This study has not been repeated, but there is no reason to doubt its continued relevance.

3. The term "managed care" is not used consistently. Some authors include bargaining for price discounts in the definition (Congressional Budget Office, 1991, 37).

to provide as few services as possible since its revenue is unaffected by how many services it provides while its costs are higher if it supplies more services. Consumers in HMOs typically pay little out-of-pocket for most services though copayments for physician visits are becoming more common. Thus, consumer demand in HMOs is high. The non-price rationing by the HMO results in lower total health care spending than those with similar 100 percent traditional insurance. The difference averages 20–30 percent. It varies with the internal organization and incentives of the HMO. Also, the mixture of services is different, with the HMOs providing much less inpatient care and slightly more outpatient care.

Other newer approaches to utilization control are less direct and sometimes less strict. One may think of them as spanning a spectrum of possibilities, with the tightly controlled HMOs at one end and traditional hands-off health insurance at the other end. On such a spectrum, PPOs are the neighbors of the HMOs. Providers contracting with PPOs agree to accommodate the PPOs' prices and utilization controls. Most PPOs require permission before a consumer is hospitalized, review whether the patient should be discharged from the hospital, and require mandatory second opinions for surgery.

Less tightly organized than the PPO is the combination of managed care with otherwise traditional insurance. Here, the control techniques are used to reduce costs, but there is no attempt to contract with selected providers.

Early examples of this type of managed care were instituted by Blue Cross of California and Oregon in response to competition by HMOs in the 1960s (Goldberg and Greenberg 1977b; 1980). But managed care in otherwise traditional insurance has grown enormously since the early 1980s. The limited research so far shows that costs are reduced by this sort of utilization control (Khandker and Manning 1992).

Managed care does not raise the financial risk facing the consumer. Conversely, it does raise the risk that the consumer will not get the medical care that he desires when he is sick because the insurer will refuse to pay for or provide it. The consumer's own preferences and values count for less under nonprice rationing. This disadvantage is held in check by competition among health insurers and providers. HMOs compete partly on the degree to which they are successful in responding to the values of their members. The HMOs, with their generally tight controls and no coverage for out-of-plan treatment, have the greatest problem accommodating a diverse population.

The disadvantage of a single HMO covering a diverse population was analyzed by Yael and Yoav Benjamini (1986, 224). They showed that a population with heterogeneous demands could be better off with traditional insurance, even compared with what they called a perfect HMO (costless and, on average, correct nonprice rationing of care).[4] The traditional insurance was subject to moral hazard, but it could accommodate diverse demands for care. Using data about employees of the University of Pennsylvania, they showed empirically that those who chose traditional insurance over the HMO were more heterogeneous in age, education, and income. The authors noted that any scheme to force all consumers into a single HMO-type scheme, like the British National Health Service, is bound to cause inefficiency. The ideal would be HMOs and other managed-care insurers competing with traditional insurers.

Competition among Medical Providers. As discussed, the type of health insurance common in the market affects competition among physicians and hospitals. Traditional insurance, by paying much of the extra cost of a higher-priced provider, reduces the incentive for consumers to search for and choose lower-priced providers. The more common this insurance is, the less providers compete. They will raise prices further above marginal costs.

Toward the other extreme, indemnity insurance leaves the difference in price between high- and low-priced providers entirely to the consumer. In this case, consumers have strong incentives to search out and choose lower-priced providers. Indemnity is thus both more efficient and more favorable to competition than insurance that pays a percentage of the bill. As a result, many economists have favored it over percentage coinsurance (Newhouse and Taylor 1970, 1971; Pauly 1971b; Frech and Ginsburg 1975, 1978b).

Preferred Provider Organizations and Competition among Providers. Going still further, PPOs can actually make the incentive to use a lower-priced provider exceed the price difference. Utilization control provides some of the cost savings of a PPO: this is not new. HMOs have been doing the same thing all along. The innovation is this: PPOs improve competition in the fee-for-service market.

The PPO improves consumer information about the low-priced providers and also strengthens the incentives for consumers to use the low-priced providers. At the same time, it improves the incentives for providers to adopt a selective low-price strategy. Consumers know

---

4. While the Benjaminis' definition of a perfect HMO is quite appropriate for their purpose, HMOs can, by responding to consumer requests, tailor their nonprice rationing to consumer values, at least to some extent.

that a certain provider has low prices simply because he is listed as a preferred provider. Further, concerns with quality are allayed because PPOs have incentives to maintain a brand name by avoiding low quality.

The PPO gives the provider a way to cut his price only to the PPO members. But even if the PPO were not to get a discount but merely to select low-price providers, it would encourage low-price providers and raise their market share. The end result is more information and better competition. Indeed, research shows PPOs obtaining discounts in the 10–20 percent range regardless of their size (Dranove, Satterthwaite, and Sindelar 1986).

The structure of PPOs provides a valuable quality control. Consumers who are unhappy with providers on the PPO's list can opt out and use nonpreferred ones. By using this safety valve, consumers police the quality of the care. If the PPO has enough data to detect that certain providers are often avoided, their performance bears review.

Health Insurance and Technological Innovation in Medicine. Health insurance also affects the direction of technological innovation because it affects the way in which providers, especially hospitals, compete. This, in turn, affects the incentive for invention and diffusion of new technology.[5]

Traditional insurance, especially if consumer copayments are low or nonexistent, shifts competition from price largely into nonprice dimensions. In such an industry, technological innovations that raised quality or convenience would be welcomed by providers regardless of cost. Conversely, innovations that cut costs, without affecting or slightly reducing quality or convenience, would be of little interest. Thus, with complete traditional insurance, quality-enhancing innovations would likely be pursued and succeed while cost-reducing ones would not.

At the opposite extreme, if no one had insurance at all, providers would compete more intensely on price. In this market, cost-reducing innovations would likely be pursued and succeed. Quality-enhancing innovations would succeed only if consumers judged the quality improvement to be worth the extra expense.

Newhouse (1978b, 1988) used this argument to explain why

---

5. For an alternative explanation involving monopoly nonprofit hospitals facing no competition, see Martin Feldstein (1971b). For a nontechnical version, see Feldstein (1971a). In this analysis, more complete health insurance simply loosens the budget constraint facing nonprofit hospital decision makers so that they can spend more on costly, prestigious new technology.

higher *levels* of hospital insurance coverage are correlated with higher *growth rates* of hospital expenses. The higher levels of insurance shift the invention and adoption of new technology in the direction of quality-enhancement, even at substantially higher cost. This raises the growth rate of hospital costs.

The Blue Cross/Blue Shield System

In the 1930s and 1940s, health care providers created the Blue Shield physician services and Blue Cross hospital services insurance companies. Still the most powerful health insurers, they are now losing some of their market share and market power (Frech and Ginsburg 1988). The various Delta Dental Plans, started by the local dental societies and generally still controlled by them, closely parallel the Blue Shield plans of the physicians. The same is true of the Vision Service Plans, organized and controlled by the optometrists. Organized health care providers created their own health insurers for many reasons, discussed below.

Expand Insurance. When the Blue plans were formed, an apparent social benefit of risk spreading was not being performed by private insurance. Most private insurers seemed to believe, incorrectly, that health care was so subject to moral hazard that it could not be reliably insured.

Raise Demand. Health insurance and health care are strong complements in demand. As we have seen, more insurance raises demand for health care. Thus, providers would like to see more insurance because it would raise demand for their services (Frech 1979, 1980a; Frech and Ginsburg 1978a; Leffler 1983). This would raise physicians' incomes. Some writers point to the problem of avoiding bad debts as a reason for the providers to establish and promote health insurers. Distinguishing this from simply raising demand is purely semantic.

There are also altruistic and philosophical motivations for raising demand. The medical societies and hospital associations created the Blue Cross and Blue Shield insurers during and immediately after the Great Depression. At that time, many consumers who ordinarily could have paid for their medical care could not or would not. In this environment, many saw the extension of health insurance to the working middle and upper classes as a charitable act even if it could not be extended to the poor or the unemployed.

On philosophical grounds, some believe that there should be no financial barriers to (consumer copayments for) health care, even for middle-class and wealthy consumers. This philosophy was and is important to the founders and decision makers of the Blue Shield and Blue Cross insurers (Berman 1978).

Note the difference between general opposition to price rationing and the belief that one should subsidize health care for the poor. The latter view, clearly explained by Pauly (1971a), is almost universally held. But this view does not imply nonmarket health care allocation.

Discouragement of Competition. Another motive for providers to promote health insurance was to avoid types of insurance that promotes competition among providers. As discussed, providers have consistently tried to suppress HMOs and PPO–type insurer contracting and also insurer utilization controls. The Blue Cross and Blue Shield plans structured their benefits and other aspects of their business to attenuate competition among physicians and hospitals.

Complete insurance (low copayment). The Blue Cross and Blue Shield plans favor comprehensive health insurance, with its tendency to reduce search and competition. The Blue Cross symbol and name were first used in 1934 by the St. Paul plan and quickly caught on with the other plans (Anderson 1975, 36). The American Hospital Association soon formed the Council on Hospital Service Plans. As early as 1938, it adopted approval principles including service benefits (100 percent, first-dollar coverage) and the idea that the plans should not compete with each other (Anderson 1975, 40).

In 1954, the Blue Cross plans assigned at least some of their rights in the Blue Cross trademark to the American Hospital Association. The agreement included several requirements that reduced the degree of competition among hospitals. Every hospital was supposed to be given a reasonable opportunity to contract with its local plan, and consumers were to have free choice among contracting hospitals. These requirements prevented the sort of competitive contracting used by PPOs and contract medicine. Benefits, ideally at 100 percent of costs, were to be provided (*Agreement between American Hospital Association and the Blue Cross Plans* 1954, 5).

The situation was similar for Blue Shield, though unlike Blue Cross and the American Hospital Association, Blue Shield's national association was never controlled directly by the American Medical Association. The earliest precursors of the Blue Shield plans were the county service bureaus set up by county medical societies in Washington State to discourage contract medicine in the 1930s. By 1937, the state medical societies of California, Michigan, and Pennsylvania had set up similar plans. By 1946, there were forty-three physician service plans nationally. In that year, the AMA contributed $25,000 to help start the Associated Medical Care Plan, which was to become the analogue of the Blue Cross Commission (Anderson 1975, 54). The Blue Shield symbol and name were first used by the Western New York Medical Plan of Buffalo. By 1947, many plans across the nation were using the symbol and name. In that year, the Blue Shield plans assigned at least some of their trademark rights to the Blue Shield Commission (*Agreement Relating to the Collective Service Mark "Blue Shield"* 1951, 1).

Blue Cross and Blue Shield membership standards. The membership standards of the national sanctioning bodies of both Blue Shield and Blue Cross are fascinating. They reflect the extra pressure in the direction of making the benefits more complete and in preventing selective contracting.

From early on, both plans required that consumers be given free choice of provider and that all providers be given a chance to contract (*Blue Cross Plan Approval Program of the American Hospital Association* 1946, 7; *Membership Standards of the National Association of Blue Shield Plans*, 13). This idea was reinforced by a requirement that the majority of providers, accounting for 75 percent of the patient days and 51 percent of the physicians, should contract with the relevant Blue Plan (*Blue Cross Plan Approval Program of the American Hospital Association* 1946, 11; *National Association of Blue Shield Plans* 1976, 13). These provisions eliminated the possibility of selective contracting, a key procompetitive element in HMO and PPO contracts.

Competition among hospitals for the right to contract with Blue Cross was virtually eliminated and collusion in general encouraged by a requirement that Blue Cross bargain with the state or local hospital organization rather than individual hospitals (*Blue Cross Plan Approval Program of the American Hospital Association* 1946, 10, 11). Blue Cross hospital rates were not to take effect unless approved by a majority (later changed to 75 percent) of the hospitals, accounting for 75 percent or more of patient days (*Blue Cross Plan Approval Program of the American Hospital Association* 1946, 11; *Approval Program for Blue Cross Plans* 1964, 7).

The approval programs were also clear in promoting the use of complete insurance. Both required that the plans offer at least one policy with 100 percent coverage. The Blue Shield standards also expressed preference for the "usual, customary and reasonable" (UCR) system and required "professional involvement" in the system's implementation (*Blue Cross Association* 1981, 1; *National Association of Blue Shield Plans* 1976, 14).

110

Blue Cross standards were quite specific on completeness of coverage. The plans were to cover not less than 75 percent of hospital bills, and they were to work toward comprehensive coverage (*Approval Program for Blue Cross Plans* 1964, 3, 5).

The "usual" or most-favored-nation clause. One of the ways that the Blue Cross/Blue Shield plans discourage competition among physicians and hospitals is their use of the "usual" component of their "usual, customary and reasonable" plans for physician services or parallel features for hospital insurance. The concept of usual prohibits selective price discounting to other insurers or to those with no insurance. It is identical to the most-favored-nation or best-price clause sometimes used in other industries.

Under the usual clause, if a provider offers a discount to a PPO or an HMO, he must offer the same price to the Blue Cross or Blue Shield plan. This contractual clause reduces the incentives for price reductions.

If the insurer using the most-favored-nation policy had a small market share, the anticompetitive effect would be likewise slight. At the same time, the policy would economize on bargaining and information costs. Thus, the use of the clause by an insurer with a small market share would probably not interfere enough with competition to be a cause for concern.[6]

The dampening effect on price competition among providers is obviously stronger the larger the local Blue Cross/Blue Shield plan's market share. Further, by weakening the ability of other insurers to channel members to price-cutting providers, most-favored-nation clauses reduce the extent of competition among health insurers. As a result, this usual or most-favored-nation clause also keeps the Blue Cross/Blue Shield market share higher.[7] The usual rule eliminates price discrimination, which is generally believed to undermine pricing

---

6. Most-favored-nation pricing clauses are used in many other industries with other interpretations, including procompetitive ones. The clause, for example, can allow a durable goods monopolist to commit not to undermine his own monopoly in the future by flooding the market (Butz 1990). Alternatively, a seller in a bilateral monopoly can avoid future bargaining about prices by using the most-favored-nations clause to tie his price to those observed in more competitive areas (Mulherin 1986).

7. The effect of most-favored-nation pricing clauses in reducing the intensity of price competition has been studied in the theoretical industrial organization literature. For game theoretic approaches see Jean Tirole (1988, 330–32), Steven C. Salop (1986, 275–78) or Charles Holt and David Scheffman (1987). For an early verbal statement of the argument, see Paul Cook (1963, 70–72).

discipline in oligopoly (Scherer 1980, 323, 324).

Blue Cross/Blue Shield plans vary in the extent to which they enforce the usual clause. Many simply ignore it. If this were not true, the
explosive growth of Independent Practice Association (IPA) HMOs
and PPOs in recent years could not have occurred.[8] But some plans do
enforce the usual clause.

The Ocean State *antitrust case.* Blue Cross/Blue Shield of Rhode
Island recently used a most-favored-nation policy to prevent hospitals
from granting discounts larger than the Blue Cross discount to Ocean
State Physicians Health Plan, a local HMO (*Ocean State v. Blue Cross
and Blue Shield of Rhode Island* 1988, 60). At the same time, it applied the
same policy against Rhode Island physicians who offered discounts to
Ocean State. The result was a massive resignation of these physicians
from Ocean State.

In the antitrust trial that ensued, the jury found Blue Cross/Blue
Shield guilty of violating section 2 (monopolization) of the Sherman
Antitrust Act and of the common law offense of interference with contractual relations (*Ocean State* 1988, 63). Judge Francis J. Boyle over-
ruled both jury verdicts, partly on technical legal grounds and partly
on the basis of a bizarre interpretation of the economics of the case.

The jury was plainly confused about the proper way to award
damages. It first tried to award damages to the physician class and to
Ocean State without tying them to specific claims. It finally awarded
damages solely for contractual interferences. The judge interpreted
this as meaning that "the jury's award of no damages on the antitrust
claims indicates that they found that the Plaintiffs were not damaged
by an antitrust violation" (Ocean State 1988, 66). The judge therefore
reasoned that there was no antitrust violation. His reasoning does not
hold up. The same actions were the basis of both claims. Thus, award-
ing damages for either claim implies that the plaintiffs were hurt by
the defendant's actions. Any allocation of damages between the two
claims would be arbitrary and meaningless.

Judge Boyle agreed that Blue Cross/Blue Shield had market
power. He also apparently accepted the testimony of Ronald Battista,
Blue Cross/Blue Shield's senior vice president of professional relations, that the most-favored-nation policy was not designed to produce
savings for Blue Cross. Also, he agreed that its most-favored-nation

---

8. As Mark Pauly (1988b) noted, the use of the most-favored-nation clause
also exacerbates the problems caused by Blue Cross/Blue Shield monopsony
power.

policy caused a large number of physicians to resign from Ocean State and therefore to stop competitive discounting of their fees. Somehow Judge Boyle then argued that the policy did not reduce competition among physicians (*Ocean State* 1988, 45). Equally incredibly, he maintained that antitrust law cannot deny a business practice to a firm with market power and permit the practice for competitors without market power (*Ocean State* 1988, 71). It is well known that the same policy can have different effects and flow from different intent depending on whether the firm has market power. Under Judge Boyle's strange doctrine, antitrust policy is supposed to ignore this difference.[9] The case seems a clear case of an insurer with market power using a most-favored-nation clause to harm competition.

The California Dental Service (Delta Dental). The usual clause has been strictly enforced by the California Dental Service (CDS), the Delta Dental plan for California. In a clear attempt to thwart the growth of price discounting to dental HMOs and PPOs, it issued the following statement:

> *Dentists who participate in* Preferred Provider Organizations (PPOs) *should be aware* that if the fees they offer through a PPO are lower than their accepted fees on file with CDS, *the lower fees will be considered* their true *"usual"* fees by CDS. (emphasis in original) (*CDS Newsletter* September–October 1983, 1)

This clause is vigorously enforced. An earlier *CDS Newsletter* (July–August 1981, 1) announced that

> so far this year (1981) dentists in Red Bluff, Riverside, Long Beach, Los Angeles, San Jose and Oakland have had their fees lowered to *match the lowest fees* they offer in their offices.
>
> Additionally, more than *200 member dentists* recently received notification that their participation in a program under which they *accepted a schedule lower* than their filed fees as full payment had brought the usualness of *their filed fees in questions.* (emphasis in original) (*CDS Newsletter* July–August 1981, 1).

But other dental insurers, who are not controlled by dentists, do not enforce the usual definition in this way.

---

9. For other recent critiques of the courts' apparent lack of concern with most-favored-nation clauses, see Jonathan Baker (1989) and David Eisenstadt (1990).

Empirical Studies of Blue Cross/Blue Shield

For the Blues to have any effect on the health care system, they must have some monopsony power as buyers in that market. Thus, we turn first to the determinants of market power as buyers.

The Sources of Blue Cross/Blue Shield Market Power. There are two major sources of market power for the Blues. First, they have important tax and regulatory advantages (Frech 1974; Thorndike 1976; Greenspan and Vogel 1982; Arnould and DeBrock 1985; Sindelar 1986, 1988). Second, in many cases, they obtain discounts and other advantages from providers.

Tax and regulatory advantages. The Blues are usually exempt from state and local property taxes. They have been completely exempt from federal income taxes until 1986; the exemption is now only partial. In most states, these plans are exempt from state premium taxation, which is often about 2 percent of premiums. This tax advantage has declined in importance in the 1970s and 1980s as many large employers have become self-insured and have thereby avoided the premium tax, whether the group policy is administered by a Blue Cross or Blue Shield plan.

The Blues have some regulatory advantages as well. Required reserves are typically less than for commercial insurers and often are nonexistent. In some states, individual commercial insurance is regulated as to loss ratio (benefits-premiums); this procedure thereby eliminates some types of insurance with high selling costs. In some states, the Blue plans' rates are regulated as to total premiums but not loss ratio. Also, some states require open enrollment periods for the Blues. While overall the Blues are favored by regulation, the last two regulations are harmful to them and are associated with lower market shares (Frech 1974; Frech and Ginsburg 1988).

Physician and hospital discounts. The other main source of the Blues' market power is the large discount many of them receive from providers. Although other cost advantages probably accrue from the Blues' historical, intimate relationships with the providers, the discounts are likely the most important.

The discounts, which can be as large as 28 percent, are both a cause and a consequence of the Blues' market power. The discounts give them a large cost advantage, which allows them to undercut the commercial insurers and increases their market share in insurance markets. But a large Blue plan share in insurance markets allows the plan to extract a large discount in the provider market by acting as a monopsonist. Hence comes a vicious circle of causation (Frech 1988a; Pauly 1988b; 1988c).

Frech (1988a, 302–3) found a strong positive empirical relationship between the physician discount and Blue Shield market share in a sample of 17 large Blue Shield plans. The discount ranged from a high of 28.2 percent in the Massachusetts plan to 1 percent in the Chattanooga, Tennessee, plan.

Several researchers have found a similarly strong positive relationship between the size of the hospital discount and the Blue Cross market share (Feldman and Greenberg 1981; Adamache and Sloan 1983). Both teams attempted to determine the direction of causation with simultaneous equations methods, but these efforts are not successful: the data are not powerful enough to identify causation statistically.

Michael Staten, William Dunkelberg, and John Umbeck (1987) argued against the idea that the Blues have monopsony power, based on their empirical analysis of local hospital markets in Indiana. They claimed to test the Blue Cross monopsony hypothesis by regressing the difference between revenues per discharge for Blue Cross and other private insurers' on the local market (county) share of Indiana Blue Cross. The data are from 1983.

As shown by Pauly (1987a) the inference is faulty. The difference in Blue Cross and commercial payments is not a measure of Blue Cross price discrimination in buying. Under some conditions, that difference might be a measure of hospital price discrimination in favor of Blue Cross, which is related to the degree of hospital monopoly power, not Blue Cross's monopsony power. Blue Cross could depress the price of hospital care to all demanders by differing amounts in differing local markets: this effect would not be picked up by Staten, Dunkelberg, and Umbeck's variable.

Further, Indiana Blue Cross paid posted charges, just as the other insurers did. As a matter of policy, Indiana Blue Cross sought to pay exactly the same prices for hospital services as other insurers. If so, how can revenues differ? There are only two ways, neither related to price differences or to monopsony. First, Blue Cross and the other insurers may differ in the completeness of coverage (consumer copayments). Whichever insurer paid a lower percentage of the bill would pay less per discharge, with the difference made up by the patient. Second, the patients with the differing types of insurance may have differing lengths of stay and use different services per hospital stay. This is a quantity measure, not a price measure. It is closely related to the case mix of the hospital inpatients with differing insurance. Neither source of variation is related to Blue Cross monopsony power, not even to hospital monopoly power.

The connection between the discounts and Blue Cross/Blue Shield market power was foreseen by the founders of the plans and was part of the effort to prevent the Blues from competing with each other. According to Rufus Rorem (1985, 13–14), one of the founders of Blue Cross,

> Hospitals faced with the possibility of doing business with one of several Plans attempted to negotiate an agreement with the plan which imposed the least financial burden on the hospital. . . . The operation of only one Plan per service area helped the Plan obtain the participation of hospitals on terms which were favorable to the Plan and its subscribers, thereby enhancing the Plan's attractiveness in the marketplace.

At least up to some point, the discounts benefit providers as a group because the discounts allow the relatively complete Blue Cross/Blue Shield insurance to attain a larger market share and thus raise demand for services. This situation raises the entire structure of prices for all insurers, including the Blues, but the Blues continue to get the discount from the now-higher average level of prices.

The existence of the discount forces a cost disadvantage on the commercial insurers but does nothing to prevent the price level from rising (Leffler 1983; Frech 1988). In fact, in a simple regression of the Blue Shield discount on per capita health care expenditures, Frech found a positive relationship between the two (Frech 1988, 307, 308). It is instructive that in many states the founding physician or hospital groups voluntarily agreed to Blue Cross or Blue Shield discounts at the time of the organization of the plans.

The discounts can be considered a more powerful version of the most-favored-nation or usual requirement that is part of almost all Blue Cross/Blue Shield insurance. With the discount, the providers are forced to charge Blue plan members a price *below* the lowest price they charge to others.

Competition among Blue Cross/Blue Shield plans. The various Blue Cross and Blue Shield plans across the nation agree to divide markets almost perfectly. With few exceptions, the plans agree on geographical markets. Further, in most areas where there are separate Blue Cross and Blue Shield plans, they agree to divide the market on a product-line basis. Blue Cross provides insurance only for hospital services while Blue Shield provides insurance only for physician services. Arguably, this amounts to collusion under the antitrust laws (Frech and Ginsburg 1978a, 184; Frech 1980b, 263).

In fact, there have been two antitrust attacks on the collusion. Both ended in settlements allowing the local Blues to compete, one within Ohio and one within Maryland (*State of Maryland v. Blue Cross and Blue Shield Association* 1987; *Blue Cross and Blue Shield Association v. Community Mutual Insurance Company and State of Ohio*, 1987). Evolving antitrust law on the matter may sooner or later force the Blues to compete. Competition would reduce the amount of market power that individual Blue Cross and Blue Shield plans have over hospitals and physicians, which would reduce their ability to extract discounts. The vicious circle would run in reverse.

Is More Output Procompetitive? William Landes (1986) disagreed with the conclusion that Blue Cross and Blue Shield geographical and product-line collusion is anticompetitive. He agreed that the Blues' agreement allows them to promote more complete insurance; he viewed this as a procompetitive outcome. In a sense, more complete insurance is more insurance. Thus, Landes maintained that this collusion supports an increase in output; therefore it must be procompetitive (1986, 13):

> I understand that the (Blue Cross and Blue Shield) Plans generally are required (with some exceptions) to serve exclusive nonoverlapping areas as a condition of receiving a license to use the "BLUE CROSS" and "BLUE SHIELD" service marks and trade names. I believe this restriction tends to expand the output of health care financing services and, therefore, is procompetitive.

In most industries, a horizontal restriction that increased the industry output would indeed be procompetitive. But the interaction of health insurance and health care reverses the common-sense conclusion. As discussed, more complete health insurance increases moral hazard welfare losses and suppresses consumer search and therefore competition in the health care market. Further, because of the tax deductibility of health insurance payments for employers, the average middle-class consumer has insurance that is too complete, even without the Blues' influence. Because of moral hazard and its harmful effects on competition, more output in the sense of more complete insurance is not a good thing. In the traditional language of antitrust, cost control is part of the output of a health insurer. An insurer that paid more claims because of poor cost control would be considered as producing less output, not more.

Blue Cross/Blue Shield Goals. As noted by Frech and Ginsburg (1978a, 170), the presence of regulatory and tax advantages for the

Blues raises a question: Since there are apparently economies of scale in health insurance (Blair, Ginsburg, and Vogel 1975; Vogel and Blair 1975b; Frech 1976; Vogel 1977), why do the Blue Cross and Blue Shield plans not have a near monopoly of the market? Frech and Ginsburg argued (1978a, 174) that the Blues use their cost advantages to purchase, in effect, two major goods or to pursue two major institutional goals. The first is relatively complete health insurance. The second is the easy life for top decision makers, leading to administrative slack or inefficiency.

Regarding the first objective, the evidence is clear that the Blues have provided far more complete (lower copayment) insurance than do their commercial competitors (Andersen and Anderson 1970; Frech 1979; Frech 1988). As the former vice president of the Blue Cross Association, Howard Berman (1978, 191), notes:

> As a matter of philosophy, Blue Cross Plans have from the outset been committed to provision of service benefits and comprehensive coverage. This commitment . . . is one of the factors which distinguishes Blue Cross Plans from commercial insurers.

An even clearer statement was approved by the board of directors of the American Hospital Association, which at that time owned the Blue Cross trademark and licensed individual plans (American Hospital Association Board of Trustees 1960, 3, 9):

> Service benefits and hospital sponsorship compose the foundation upon which the Blue Cross prepayment program is built . . . full service benefits (which pay one hundred percent of all hospital bills) come out as the preferred method of payment. . . . Hospitals have the responsibility for . . . (the) promotion of prepayment plans which offer full service benefits.

Thus, the Blues use some of their competitive advantage to promote complete insurance (Frech 1974; Frech and Ginsburg 1978a; Landes 1986, 14, 15; Frech 1980b; Frech and Ginsburg 1988). The Blues' commitment to relatively complete insurance allows a major role for commercial insurers with more consumer copayment, even though the tax and regulatory advantages of the Blues give them artificially lower costs. Some consumers strongly prefer less complete insurance.

The pursuit of administrative slack or inefficiency is not explicit. Rather, it results from the nonprofit form of the Blues. Since they cannot pay dividends to their owners or to the hospitals and physicians who founded them, the incentive to keep costs low and to administer the firms efficiently is weaker than for the profit-seeking commercial insurers (Alchian 1961; Alchian and Kessel 1962; Williamson 1970; Alchian and Demsetz 1972). Even the mutual health insurers have better incentives because their controlling managers can effectively capture some of the residual profits or rents (Frech 1980b).

Blue Cross/Blue Shield Efficiency. There is a good deal of evidence that the Blues are, on average, less efficient than the commercial insurers. Frech (1976; 1980b) compared the costs of administering Medicare claims for Blue Shield Plans, mutual insurers, and profit-seeking insurers. Blue Shield costs were about 40 percent higher than the profit-seeking insurers', while mutual insurers' costs were about 20 percent higher. Blue Shield and the mutual firms were also inferior to the profit-seeking firms in processing speed and accuracy, even when scale of operation is controlled for.[10] These findings were confirmed by a larger-scale study by Ronald Vogel and Roger Blair (1975a, 1975b). But, using more recent data, Stephen Mennemeyer (1984) did not find a consistent cost disadvantage for the Blue Shield plans. The results of these studies differ enough that reconciling the findings would be a valuable research project.

One disadvantage of these studies is the lack of constancy for either the degree of competitive advantages of the plans or the degree of physician domination of them. Both factors were shown to matter and are discussed below.

Kuo-Cheng Tseng (1978) found Blue Cross Medicare intermediaries for hospital costs lower for some costs and higher for others compared with commercial Medicare intermediaries; the Blue Cross plans had lower administrative costs but did not report any statistics for total costs. His study may have been flawed because of analyzing costs per claim rather than per dollar processed. There is some evidence that the commercial insurers are more efficient at aggregating claims (Frech 1976). In related work, William Hsiao (1978) found Blue Cross far more efficient than the former Department of Health, Education and Welfare in administering Medicare claims.

The regulatory and tax advantages of the Blues have been statistically related to two proxies for Blue plan market power across states or plan market areas. The first is Blue Cross and Blue Shield market shares; the second is administrative costs. Since Blue Cross/Blue Shield insurance is more complete, the relationship of the regulatory advantages to the Blue market shares has been measured in the context

---

10. Most Blue Cross and Blue Shield plans are smaller than commercial insurers because of their agreement, through the national Blue Cross and Blue Shield Association, not to compete with each other. Most of the agreed market areas are states or even smaller areas.

of models of the demand for health insurance. The consistent finding is that the tax and regulatory advantages raise the market shares of the Blue plans (Frech 1974; Thorndike 1976; Frech and Ginsburg 1978a, 1981; Arnould and Eisenstadt 1981; Eisenstadt and Kennedy 1981; Feldman and Greenberg 1981; Greenspan and Vogel 1982; Adamache and Sloan 1983; Goldberg and Greenberg 1985; Sindelar 1986; Arnould and DeBrock 1985).

But the tax and regulatory advantages have been found to lead to higher Blue Plan administrative costs (Vogel and Blair 1975a, 1975b; Vogel 1977; Frech and Ginsburg 1978a, 1981; Arnould and DeBrock 1985; Eisenstadt and Kennedy 1981). Eisenstadt and Kennedy also showed that where physicians have more complete control of the local Blue Shield plan, administrative costs are lower. They reasoned that physicians can transfer cost savings to themselves in the form of higher insurance payments; thus they have good incentives to monitor the Blue Shield plans to keep costs down.

Some preliminary research by Stephen Foreman, John Wilson, and Richard Scheffler (1995), using more recent data from the 1980s, indicates that this traditional relationship may have changed as the Blue plans have lost market power and cost advantages in the emerging, more competitive health insurance markets. They found that in this more recent data higher Blue Cross/Blue Shield market shares are associated with lower administrative costs.

Blue Cross/Blue Shield Market Power Is Unusually Durable. Ordinarily, a monopsony would provide profit opportunities for competing firms. Sellers would shift from the monopsonist to other purchasers. Over time, the competing buyers would erode the underlying market power of the monopsonist. This seems to be happening only quite slowly for the Blue Cross and Blue Shield plans. The reason appears to be the all-or-nothing nature of the Blue Cross/Blue Shield offers to providers, coupled with the organization of the health care system.

A provider must agree to the Blue plan's discount or be classified as a nonparticipating provider. This differs from a PPO in that the Blue plan usually tries to contract with all or most providers. In some states with small Blue Cross or Blue Shield plans or where nonparticipating providers are paid almost the same as participating providers, this is not much of a hardship—and those states have little or no discount. But where the payment for nonparticipating providers is much less than for participating providers and where the Blues have large market shares, most physicians and hospitals appear unwilling to give up completely on the Blues' business to concentrate on those with other insurance.

Massachusetts Blue Shield is a particularly extreme example. It pays nothing to nonparticipating physicians or to their patients. At the same time, it has a large market share. Not surprisingly, it has the largest physician discounts in the United States, about 30 percent of market fees (Frech 1988). Also not surprisingly, health care costs in Massachusetts are the highest in the nation (1988).

The Effects of Blue Cross/Blue Shield Market Power. The market power of the Blues has many consequences for health care markets. Most of them promote inefficiency.

Blue Cross raises hospital costs. Those who defend the existing market power for the Blue Cross plans and their policies, such as agreeing to exclusive noncompeting market areas, make three arguments. First, Blue Cross must be a large part of the market for Blue Cross to receive the benefits of any cost control mechanisms it introduces. If utilization norms or prices decline, all insurers and the uninsured benefit. Thus, the incentive for a Blue Cross plan to introduce cost controls rises as its market share rises (Pauly 1980a, 655; Havighurst 1988, 340–42).

Second, some argue that a single insurer with a large market share would be able to use its monopsony power to drive down prices and utilization and thus effectively control price (Havighurst 1988, 236–342). This is the view of some proponents of national health insurance or some national health care reform bills: the government would play the role of the insurer with a large market share (Evans 1974; Culyer, Maynard, and Williams 1981, 147–50). Pauly (1988b, 259–60) criticized this view: he noted that an insurer with monopsony power has the incentive to depress price too far. The third argument is simpler: Blue Cross/Blue Shield must insure a large part of the provider's customers, or providers will simply ignore its cost-control efforts.

Three studies show that, on balance, these arguments are false. Where the Blue Cross market share is higher, hospital expenditures are higher. The first study illustrates the mechanism. Using data across states from 1969, Frech (1974, 1979) estimated a simultaneous equation market model determining Blue Cross market share, the average completeness of insurance, and hospital price. Higher Blue Cross market shares led to more complete insurance, measured by the average proportion of hospital bills paid by third parties. (Also, larger Blue Cross market shares were associated with smaller Blue Cross deductibles.) More complete insurance, in turn, was associated with higher demand price for hospital care. In tracing the effects through, a halving of the Blue Cross market share from 0.44 to 0.22 would reduce hospital price by 7 percent (Frech 1976, 67). In the Frech study, causation is assumed to occur only through Blue Cross affecting the completeness of insurance.

A pair of later studies impose less theoretical structure. They relate the Blue Cross market share directly to hospital prices or costs. Frech and Ginsburg (1978a) examined the effect of variations in Blue Cross market share across forty-six states, again with 1969 data. A simple reduced-form equation was estimated for both price (daily semiprivate room charges) and average cost of a bed day. The regression held constant the price of health insurance, income, the quantity of hospital care demanded, and urbanization. A higher Blue Cross market share was found to have a large effect in raising hospital prices. A halving of Blue Cross market share from its national average (in 1969) would reduce hospital prices by about 10 percent. This result was not affected by adding a variable controlling for whether the Blue Cross plan paid hospital charges or costs. It was statistically significant at about the 96 percent level on a two-tailed test. The effect on hospital costs was also positive, slightly larger in dollar terms but about half as large in percentage terms. It was statistically significant at about the 85 percent level (Frech and Ginsburg 1978a, 180–83). These results indicate that a high Blue Cross market share is associated with high hospital prices and costs.

These results were confirmed by an analysis of a larger and later data set by Joel Hay and Michael Leahy (1984). They used 1978 data, with observations of 202 Health Systems Agency regions. These regions span the country and were originally designed to comprise independent self-contained health care delivery systems. The average population contained was just over 1 million (1984, 836, 838).

Hay and Leahy held more cost and demand influences constant than did Frech and Ginsburg. Examples include hospital employee wages, physician-to-population ratios, and educational level. They found that higher Blue Cross/Blue Shield market shares and lower commercial market shares are strongly related to higher hospital (and nonhospital) utilization and costs. For the variables most comparable to the Frech and Ginsburg study, Hay and Leahy estimated that a halving of the Blue Cross/Blue Shield market share would cut hospital costs by 6 percent (identical to Frech and Ginsburg's estimate) and the incidence of surgery per admission by 7 percent (Hay and Leahy 1984, 838–42).[11]

A high market share for the Blues is strongly related to high costs

---

11. This calculation assumes that the Blues lose market share to commercial insurers. The estimates are somewhat higher if one assumes that they lose market share to HMOs.

and prices for health care, at least through the early 1980s. Whatever the Blues claim about their administrative cost controls, either they did not work better than the commercial insurers' cost controls, or they were not effective enough to overcome the impact of the more complete insurance promoted by the Blues. A preliminary study of Blue Cross (only) costs suggests that the past relationship may have weakened or reversed as the Blue plans have lost market power (Foreman, Wilson, and Scheffler 1995). It would be interesting to see if the earlier relationship of Blue Plan market share to the *total* cost has held up in more recent years, but the necessary Blue Cross/Blue Shield data are no longer public.

Physician Control of Blue Shield and Fees. The first empirical analysis of Blue Cross and Blue Shield costs, market share, and regulatory advantages (Frech and Ginsburg 1978a, 1981) found that it was easier to explain Blue Cross than Blue Shield costs. David Eisenstadt and Thomas Kennedy (1981) argued that the problems in modeling Blue Shield behavior came from ignoring variations in the extent of physician control among the Blue Shield plans. They contended that where physicians dominate the plans, they have a strong incentive to keep costs down. Physicians can transfer wealth from the Blue Shield plans to themselves by paying higher fees. Thus, the physicians are residual claimants, like the stockholders of the typical profit-seeking firm.

The empirical results are consistent with this view. Eisenstadt found that, holding market variables constant, a higher percentage of physicians on the Blue Shield board of directors lowered costs. For Blue Shield plans with tax advantages, a 10 percent increase in the proportion of physicians on the board reduced costs by about 0.7 percent (of premiums). For Blue Shield plans without the tax advantage, the effect was about half as large.

Richard Arnould and Lawrence DeBrock (1985) confirmed this result in both a reduced form analysis and in a simultaneous equations model determining Blue Shield market share, operating costs, surgical fees, and surgical utilization. The data were cross-sectional by Blue Shield plan for 1975 and 1976.

On the matter of physician control of Blue Shield and physician fees, there is some controversy. Clearly, local Blue Shield plans have some market power that would allow them to pay supracompetitive fees, to physicians. A great deal of work has been done on the connection of physician control of Blue Shield to physician fees. Part of the impetus to this work originated in a Federal Trade Commission investigation into the issue of physician control. FTC staff lawyers found that physician control tended to raise physician prices (Stone et al. 1979,

125–90) and recommended that an FTC rule be promulgated prohibiting a physician organization from controlling or participating in controlling a Blue Shield plan (1979, 314, 315).

Underlying this staff report and recommendation was an empirical analysis by FTC economists David Kass and Paul Pautler (1981). They found that more physician control, as measured either by medical society control or by the percentage of physicians on the board of directors of the plan, led to higher maximum customary allowed fees under the Blue Shield plans' "usual, customary and reasonable" (UCR) physician reimbursement.[12, 13] The data were cross-sectional over plan areas for 1973–1977. The effect of medical society control was found to be larger than the effect of more physicians on the board of directors. They did not find that physician control influenced costs, but they did not interact physician control with regulatory or tax advantages.

Some versions of this model included a dummy variable for a merger of the Blue Cross and Blue Shield plans and a continuous variable for the size of the Blue Cross hospital discount. Such a merger raises the possibility that the physicians can profit from Blue Cross's market power as well as Blue Shield's and can therefore raise fees further. These variables were generally statistically significant.

Using the maximum customary allowable payment under Blue Shield as the dependent variable creates a problem. The connection of the maximal allowance to average fees can be quite weak. Further, Blue Shield, through a combination of complete insurance and a discount, can raise the fees charged to other insurers without necessarily raising the fees allowed in its own payments. Thus, using the maximum customary payment may miss the main effect of Blue Shield market power influence on provider fees.

Arnould and Eisenstadt (1981) and Arnould and DeBrock (1985) corroborated the Kass and Pautler studies, but used an index of the actual level of charges for surgical services. They found that physician, and especially medical society, control of Blue Shield plans was associated with higher surgical fees charged to all insurers. They found that physician control raised fees substantially more in areas where

---

12. The UCR system might seem to be outside the control of the Blue Shield plan. But the insurer controls the frequency of updates, the percentile used, whether specialists are treated differently, and whether there is a usual profile for the individual physician. Further, discounts of varying sizes are built into most Blue Shield UCR systems.

13. Maximum customary fees are the highest fees allowed under the system. They are not affected by the individual physician's usual fees and any limits that may result from them.

the Blue Shield plan had greater tax advantages over its commercial competitors. They did not include a variable for Blue Shield/Blue Cross merger.

William Lynk (1981) supplied the controversy on this issue. He found that physician control reduces Blue Shield–allowed fees. He rationalized this counterintuitive finding by an interesting application of public choice voting analysis. Lynk argued that each physician wants the maximum allowable charge to be equal to his own charge but not above it. This ensures that his fee is covered but weakens competition from physicians who charge more. If we view the medical society as operating by simply majority voting, with no side payments or logrolling, then it suffices to examine the preferences of the median physician. Thus, a medical society–controlled Blue Shield plan would want to see its maximum allowable fee at the fiftieth percentile. Lynk argued that consumers prefer a higher maximum customary allowance because they wish for a high probability that their insurance will cover the fees from the physician that they select. Since commercial insurers, which reflect consumer tastes without physician influence, typically use the ninetieth percentile, this seems reasonable.

Lynk noted that second-round effects, such as too low of a maximum allowance harming the Blue Shield market share, would be taken account of by the physician-voters (1981, 162). But still, he argued, the direction of influence would be physician control to lead to lower allowances, not higher ones.

Lynk, however, ignored another second-round effect, one that is probably more important. Physicians are concerned about the effect of the maximum allowance on competition among physicians. In particular, if the allowance is set low, the higher-priced, higher-quality physicians have an incentive to reduce their prices to compete with the lower-priced physicians. Thus, in considering feedback effects increasing the degree of competition among physicians, even the median physician may want the maximum allowance set above his fees and, in fact, higher than consumers would like.

Lynk tested his predictions empirically. First, he estimated simple reduced form equations determining the average level of Blue Shield reimbursement actually paid for forty-five procedures under the federal employees high-option plan. Payment was on a UCR basis. The observations were Blue Shield plans and procedures. Dummy variables were entered to control for procedure. Lynk found a small but statistically significant effect: physician control tended to reduce the average reimbursement. A 10 percent increase in the physicians on the board reduced the average reimbursement by about 1.5 percent. While this

125

analysis used a different dependent variable, it contradicts the other work.

Second, more closely parallel to the analysis of Kass and Pautler, Lynk estimated equations determining the maximum customary allowance over Blue Shield plans. Here, he pooled sixteen or eighteen procedures, depending on the data source. Again, he found a small negative effect of physician control. This is strongly statistically significant in all but one equation.

Specification of the equations between Lynk and Kass and Pautler show several differences. The main one is the variable for whether the Blue Cross and Blue Shield plan is merged; this variable was excluded by Lynk. Lynk stated that this exclusion was the main cause of the differences (1981, 171, 172). Also Lynk included the Blue Shield market share and treated it as exogenous. Further, Lynk pooled sixteen or eighteen procedures, while Kass and Pautler pooled only five. Pooling procedures can easily create econometric problems. In particular, pooling can cause overstatements of the accuracy of one's results. Kass and Pautler limited their pooling because the standard test for the appropriateness of pooling was violated when they included more procedures.

Just for scale reasons, the residuals or errors for the more costly procedures will be much larger and lead to heteroskedasticity. More serious, there are probably strong correlations in errors across procedures for each plan. That is, a plan that pays a relatively high amount for one procedure is more likely to do the same for others. Failing to take account of these correlations will overstate the accuracy of one's results. Each procedure gets equal weight regardless of how common it is. A quantity-weighted price index, such as used by Arnould and DeBrock, avoids this problem. Lynk ignored the degree of tax advantage of the Blue Shield plan, which the work of Arnould and Eisenstadt (1981) and Arnould and DeBrock (1985) found important.

Further, a Blue Shield plan might decrease competition overall and thus raise fees, while keeping its own payments low through the Blue Shield discount. A better dependent variable is fees charged to all insurers, not average or maximum Blue Shield reimbursements. Arnould and Eisenstadt (1981) and Arnould and DeBrock (1985) used this measure.

In their preliminary work, Foreman, Wilson, and Scheffler (1995) took a completely different approach; they used more recent data and found that higher Blue Cross/Blue Shield market share was associated with lower payments to providers (hospitals and physicians aggregated) and also with lower premiums. It will be interesting to see if more definitive versions get the same results.

The paper of Arnould and DeBrock is the most convincing. More physician control probably leads to higher fees. But an analysis reconciling Lynk's work with the other studies would be of real value. Both the tax advantages of the Blue Shield plan and whether it has merged with the Blue Cross plan are probably important. They both indicate more monopoly rents that the Blue Shield plan might transfer to physicians by increasing their fees. Still, it is troubling that the results are sensitive to such apparently minor differences in specification.

Blue Cross/Blue Shield Market Power and Open Enrollment. Open enrollment periods allow consumers to purchase insurance on an individual (nongroup) basis, regardless of health status or preexisting conditions. Though the practice is becoming rare, some Blue Cross and Blue Shield plans offer open enrollment or lax underwriting for individuals with a high risk of high health care costs. This performs a charitable function since without insurance at least some of these consumers would rely on public or private charitable care. Open enrollment is one of the rationales for the Blues' tax and regulatory advantages.

Early Blue Cross and Blue Shield plans practiced community rating, wherein all consumers paid the same premiums regardless of health status or recent experience. (Rates may differ for such easily observable features as age and sex.) In the early days of the Blues, known high-risk consumers were often allowed to purchase insurance at the community rate (Fanara and Greenberg 1985, 185–86; U.S. General Accounting Office 1986, 1–3; MacIntyre 1962).

Community rating requires market power. The insurer must set prices above costs for the relatively low risks to earn monopoly rents. These monopoly rents are used to subsidize the insurance for the high risks. Under increasing competition from the commercial insurers, the Blues dropped community rating for groups almost completely as early as 1960 (MacIntyre 1962).

Increasing competition from commercial insurers, HMOs, and PPOs has reduced the ability of Blues to subsidize health insurance for high-risk individuals. Also, regulation holding down the premiums that the Blues may charge to individuals restricts their ability and willingness to subsidize high-risk individuals. Over time, both have occurred. The result has been investigated by the U.S. General Accounting Office (1986). Researchers took 129 known high-risk test cases insured to six Blue plans and five commercial insurers. A surprising 67 percent of them were offered commercial insurance by one of the five firms. Three of the Blues charged special higher rates for high-risk individuals (if they were willing to insure them at all); the insurance offered to high-risk individuals was less complete than ordinary individual insurance, often excluding the high-risk medical conditions from the policies.

Of the six Blue Cross/Blue Shield plans investigated, two (Maryland and New York) offered continuous open enrollment, one (District of Columbia) offered annual one-month open enrollment periods, and three did not offer open enrollment of any kind (California, Connecticut, and Illinois). Survey research showed that only fifteen Blue Cross/Blue Shield plans offered open enrollment (U.S. General Accounting Office 1986, 2). The GAO concluded that the treatment of high-risk individuals by the Blues and the commercials was similar and that this analysis diminished the "justification of the plans' (federal) tax exempt status" (U.S. General Accounting Office 1986, 20). Subsequently, in the Tax Reform Act of 1986, Congress imposed a small federal income tax on the Blues.

The effect of both competition and regulation on the enrollment of nongroup consumers in Blue plans has been investigated by Philip Fanara and Warren Greenberg (1985), with cross-sectional data for 1979. They found that enrollment of nongroup consumers was lower where there was more competition from HMOs and where the Blues' nongroup rates were regulated.

Nonprofit monopoly. A special danger apparently exists in nonprofit monopoly. It may persist in imposing its philosophy on the market because it is partially insulated from the judgment of consumers expressed in the market. A profit-seeking monopoly, conversely, has strong incentive to cater to consumer demands and values so that it can earn more profits. Though perhaps slightly dulled by the lack of product market competition, these incentives are stronger than those of a nonprofit monopoly. Even though managed by public-spirited citizens, a nonprofit monopoly may be more harmful to consumers than an ordinary profit-seeking one.

The Decline of Blue Cross/Blue Shield Market Power

In the past decade or so, the Blue Cross/Blue Shield plans have lost some of their market power. There are a number of reasons for this.

Tax Advantages. The tax advantages of the Blues have declined in many states and also at the federal level. This has partly been in response to the growing perception that the public service activities of the Blues, primarily enrolling high-risk individuals at lower than competitive rates, are actually quite limited (U.S. General Accounting Office 1986).

Physician and Hospital Discounts. The other main source of Blue advantage, the physician and hospital discount, has also been eroding. This has happened partly through state governmental action. State hospital rate regulation has typically cut the Blue Cross discount. The political forces for this are probably similar to those reducing the Blues' tax advantages.

Employer Self-Insurance. Last, more and more large groups are retaining the risk of their health insurance themselves and contracting out to administrative service only (ASO) organizations (often Blue Cross/Blue Shield plans). This practice is misleadingly called self-insurance. Self-insurance gives employers several advantages by avoiding state insurance regulation. Perhaps most important, it allows groups to avoid state-mandated coverage rules that would otherwise force them to add expensive and unpopular coverage. A "self-insuring" group avoids state premium taxation.

Competition among the Blue Plans. The last element is just emerging. As discussed, the Blue plans are moving to competition with each other. Settlements of antitrust suits have led to competition among Ohio plans and also, in Maryland, between the District of Columbia and Maryland plans (Frech and Ginsburg 1988, 285). This competition will force the Blues to be more sensitive to the demands and values of the customers and allow them less latitude in imposing their own vision of overly complete insurance on the market.

Consumer Choice of Insurance Plan

For various reasons, it is valuable to know how consumers choose their health insurance plan, especially which plans compete most closely with each other. Since most American health insurance is provided by employment groups, there are two levels of choice.

The first choice is made by the employer (or perhaps the union). This is the choice of how many and which plans to offer to employees. Mark Pauly and Gerald Goldstein (1976) have examined this choice theoretically and empirically. They found a price elasticity of demand, by the group, for additional insurance of about -2.0. Interestingly, they found a positive income elasticity among unionized employment groups but a small negative income elasticity among nonunionized groups. Choice and competition at this level seem more important than

129

choice and competition in the plans offered to the group.

The second level of choice is the choice of the employees among the options given by the employer. This is of policy interest for at least two reasons. First, federal law is designed to encourage the choice of HMOs over conventional insurance. Second, for antitrust purposes, it is important to know which kinds of insurers are close competitors to each other and which are not.

Tentatively, different kinds of health insurance schemes apparently are surprisingly poor substitutes in demand for each other. Employees are not willing to switch to a different kind of insurer, such as from a conventional insurer to an HMO, in response to small price differences. They are only a bit more willing to switch from low-option conventional insurer to a high-option one with fuller coverage (Feldman, Dowd, Finch, and Cassou 1989; Short and Taylor 1989). Short and Taylor found that the price elasticity of choice of a high-option insurance plan was only about -0.14. The elasticity of choice of an HMO was even lower, at -0.07 (304, 307).

Apparently, insurers of different types are not close enough substitutes to much constrain each others' pricing. Thus, insurers of different types would be in different, though related, markets for antitrust purposes. This finding is also consistent with the work of Gail Jensen and Michael Morrisey (1990), who used a hedonic approach to see the relative values consumers placed on different aspects of health insurance plans.

In sum, health insurance competition has powerful effects on health care markets. More competitive health insurance markets lead to more efficient and more competitive health services markets.

7
Adverse Selection

Adverse selection occurs when consumers know more about their expected health expenses than the insurance sellers know or can find out (Pauly 1974a, 44–45; 1986, 649; Akerlof 1970; Rothschild and Stiglitz 1976). In this situation of asymmetric information, if the high- and low-risk consumers are pooled, the prices charged for the insurance cannot perfectly reflect the degree of risk. The prices to the low risks will be too high, while the prices to the high risks will be too low. With this inaccurate pricing, the high risks are more likely to purchase insurance than are the low risks. Thus, the selection of consumers who purchase the insurance is not random; it is adverse. If there is an equilibrium under adverse selection, the high risks will purchase the optimal amount of insurance, and good risks too little. It is also possible that the equilibrium or even the market itself fails to exist. The results of adverse selection can range from disastrous to negligible, depending on the situation.

Adverse selection occurs on unobservable characteristics. If older consumers or females choose more complete insurance or avoid HMOs, this is not adverse selection. Since the characteristics are observable, the insurer or group could adjust the rates to reflect the risks. Information is not asymmetric.

While adverse selection ordinarily is discussed in terms of purchasing similar insurance, it is also possible when the insurance contracts differ by type. Some observers claim that HMOs benefit from favorable selection when they compete with traditional third-party insurance because they attract younger consumers.

But age is observable and ratable, thus not even a logical candidate for adverse selection. HMOs do appeal disproportionately to the young because younger consumers are less likely to have a permanent relationship with one or more fee-for-service physicians. Thus, the young are less concerned about being restricted to HMO member physicians. Similarly, HMOs also appeal more to those who have recently moved to a new city because they economize on search costs. Movers are disproportionately young and healthy.

A favoring of HMOs by the young has been documented, for example, by Joachim Neipp and Richard Zeckhauser (1985). They examined the choices of Harvard University employees between HMOs and traditional Blue Cross/Blue Shield insurance. As is common, the employees' payment to the health insurer did not depend on age. Thus, 68.5 percent of employees with ten years or less of service chose an HMO, while only 32.4 percent of those with eleven years or more chose them (Neipp and Zeckhauser 1985, 66). Conversely, Susan Hosek, M. Susan Marquis, and Kenneth Wells (1991) found no favorable selection into PPOs.

The Effects of Adverse Selection

First, the market can fail to exist. That is, no firm will be willing to sell insurance at any price. Second, equilibrium may exist. If so, it separates the consumers according to their risk classes. This creates no problems for the high risks. They can buy optimal insurance and pay the expected costs of the insurance. The low risks are left with less complete insurance. Third, the market can exist, but equilibrium does not exist: any distribution of insurance plans could be altered by new entrants. These three situations will be examined.

The Market Does Not Exist. If adverse selection is severe enough, all insurance contracts can lose money. At low rates, too many high risks buy insurance; therefore the insurer loses money. As the insurer tries to avoid losses by raising prices, the better risks are driven out. If this happens fast enough as price rises, perhaps there is no price where the insurer can break even, hence no market.

It is easier to see the problem in the used car or "lemons" market, as first shown by George Akerlof (1970). The sellers of used cars are in the position of the insurance customers, with better information about their cars than buyers have. The buyers of the cars are in the position of the insurers. Suppose that buyers cannot see the quality of automobiles, but there are two kinds: good ones and bad ones (lemons). Suppose the price started out reflecting the value of the good cars. This is a high price for a lemon, so all lemons will be offered. Some good cars also will be offered. As buyers learn that they are getting some lemons, they will offer less for the cars, as a reflection of the mixture of good cars and lemons being offered. The reduction in price will drive some good cars off the market and none of the lemons. (The price is still more than a lemon is worth.) If the dropping price drives out enough of the good cars, eventually all the good cars will be driven from the market.

This radical outcome seems true for recent, late-model used cars, which are rarely traded. When they are traded, the price is much less than the price of new cars.

Separating Equilibrium May Exist. Separating equilibrium can be best analyzed in a simple model constructed by Michael Rothschild and Joseph Stiglitz (1976). Their model includes two risk classes: high and low. The low risks value any insurance contract lower than the high risks. This is also true for the additional insurance offered by a more complete policy over a less complete policy.

Thus, let us start with a situation where a single insurer offers a policy that pools the high and low risks. This cannot be an equilibrium. Another insurer can design a policy that is less complete and cheaper and attracts only the lower risks. This leaves the first insurer with high risks only; therefore he loses money. Pooling both high and low risks in one insurance policy cannot be an equilibrium.

After entry, the first insurer can raise the price of his policy for the high risks up to the breakeven point. The insurer covering the low risk can offer more complete insurance, up to the point where the high risks are indifferent between the two policies. Thus, it is the decisions of the high risks that keep the insurance coverage of the low risks less complete. If the insurer of the low risks were inadvertently to attract the high risks, he would lose money.

This separating equilibrium creates no problem for the high risks. They can get optimal insurance, and they pay competitive rates for it. For the higher risk, the adverse selection outcome is the same as if there was no adverse selection. The low risks do not fare so well. Their best choice is less complete insurance than they could choose if information on their riskiness were perfect. This less complete insurance is nonetheless competitively priced.[1]

The Market Exists, but Equilibrium Does Not. The separating equilibrium just described may not exist. Possibly no combinations of rates and insurance benefit structures allow insurers to break even and cannot be invaded by entrants offering different benefits. In such a situation, new contracts can always attract some good risks away and cause losses for the original insurers. If so, we say that there is not equilibrium.

This point is convenient to discuss in the Rothschild and Stiglitz framework. Suppose that a combination of policies that looks like the separating equilibrium is in place. If there are few high-risk consumers

---

1. If the low-risk consumers differ in tastes, some will take the more complete insurance even at high prices, and some will take no insurance at all.

in the total pool, a third insurer can offer a pooling package that is favored by all consumers—and thus destroys the previous potential equilibrium. We have already shown that the pooling package cannot be an equilibrium either. Another new entrant can pick off the good risks with a different, less complete benefit structure.

The empirical implications of this lack of equilibrium cannot be derived from the model itself. Mark Pauly has argued that the nonexistence of equilibrium would lead to instability in which relatively complete insurance would disappear and then reappear (1986, 650–51). As he noted, neither this nor any other kind of instability has been observed in health insurance markets.

Implications for Employee Group Management

The managers of employee groups can avoid most of the ill effects of adverse selection by the careful choice of plans and pricing. Jonathan Cave (1985) and Rothschild and Stiglitz (1976) have shown that within a group a cross-subsidy from the low risks to the high risks can improve welfare for all members.

To see this, remember that the low-risk employees' insurance is constrained to be so incomplete that it is not chosen by the high-risk employees. Thus, a subsidy of the more complete policy chosen by the high-risk workers discourages them from shifting to the policy favored by the low risks. This situation allows the policy for the low risks to be more complete without attracting the high risks.

This cross-subsidy requires control of pricing and prevention of entry. The cross-subsidy suggested by the theory is observed in groups with choices of plans (Farley and Monheit 1985, 232).

A simpler approach is for the group to offer only one plan. This approach completely avoids adverse selection within the group. Indeed, offering only one plan is the most common employer decision. Offering only one plan necessarily ignores differences among consumers in tastes, location, and so on. With only one plan, employees are more likely to choose no insurance. Allowing consumers to choose different plans because of differing tastes, for example, for risk, is beneficial.

While superficially it might appear to be anticompetitive for the employer or group manager to offer only one policy, this is not so. There are two possible decisions, thus two possible points where competition occurs. First, competition can be chosen by the employer; second, competition can be chosen by the employee from the menu offered by the employer. Competition to be chosen by the employer is more important; this point appears to have been missed by Enthoven

(1978, 1988, 1993), who favors forcing employers to offer three or more different insurance plans.

Empirical Evidence on Adverse Selection

There is little direct evidence on how important adverse selection is in health insurance because moral hazard also is common in health care and it is often hard to disentangle the two empirically, though they are conceptually distinct. Utilization, for example, is usually higher for those choosing a high-option over a low-option health insurance. But that would be expected from the effect of moral hazard alone. Evidence for moral hazard requires that the difference in utilization exceed that expected from moral hazard alone. Such large differences have not been found.

But, if adverse selection were a major problem in health insurance, it would have some strong empirical implications. We should observe that those who choose no insurance or less incomplete insurance (high coinsurance, deductibles, indemnity features), holding constant their access to insurance, would have better mortality and morbidity experience than those with insurance.[2] The uninsured should also use less health care. These differences should be large because the uninsured and less completely insured also would face less or no moral hazard subsidy effect from their insurance. Thus, moral hazard and adverse selection would work in the same direction to exaggerate the differences in health care use. Adverse selection has sometimes been claimed as the cause of growth in the percentage of consumers with no health insurance.

The Growth in the Uninsured. The number of uninsured has grown during the 1980s: from 12.2 percent in 1978 to 15.7 percent in 1989 (Congressional Budget Office 1991, 67, n. 2). Some observers have blamed this on an increase in adverse selection in individual insurance markets (Enthoven 1988, 44). The increase in adverse selection, in turn, has been tied to increasing competition in insurance markets (Fuchs 1986, 353). But this explanation is not convincing: some facts do not fit.

Some uninsured are full-time workers in large or medium-size firms, where they are offered group insurance. Fully 67.6 percent of

---

2. As an approximation, one could restrict comparisons to those who could not buy insurance through their employers. Presumably these consumers would have had identical opportunities to purchase individual (nongroup) insurance in the market. Some variables representing local market opportunities (such as city size) might be held constant as well.

the uninsured are full-time workers or their dependents. More than half of the uninsured employees work for large (twenty-five or more employees) firms, which usually offer health insurance (70, 71).

Other causes explain the rise in the uninsured without invoking increasing adverse selection. Many states cut back on Medicaid eligibility during the 1980s. Some former Medicaid beneficiaries chose not to buy private insurance and thus swelled the ranks of the uninsured.

Some federal and state regulation of HMOs has prevented them from insuring high-risk individuals. Federally qualified HMOs, for example, are not allowed to charge high-risk individuals higher rates nor are they allowed to use waivers of coverage for preexisting conditions. Some states apply the same rule (Congressional Budget Office 1991, 71). This rule increases the number of uninsured consumers.

State insurance regulation. Inadvertently, state health insurance regulation has increased the ranks of the uninsured. In recent years, most states have mandated that certain benefits, such as mental health benefits and drug rehabilitation services, be included in any group insurance plan. Some groups and consumers did not purchase those benefits before because they did not think them worth the cost. Forcing them to purchase insurance with the mandated benefits added hits these groups like a tax and leads some groups and individuals to drop their coverage. Because these laws do not apply to employer self-insurance, they have most of their effect on the small employers who often do not offer health insurance. To encourage more employers to offer health insurance, several states have recently dropped or softened these rules to allow bare-bones or no-frills health insurance, without mandated benefits.

Two studies have shown state-mandated benefits to be a major cause of more consumers being uninsured. John Goodman and Gerald Musgrave (1988) found that mandates were responsible for 14 percent of the uninsured in 1986. Gail Jensen and Jon Gabel (1991) showed that mandates caused 20 percent of small firms (those with fewer than twenty-five employees) to decide not to offer health insurance to their employees in 1985. By 1988, mandates had become more pervasive and inclusive and caused 43 percent of small firms to decide not to offer group health insurance. Goodman (1991) argued that other detailed state regulations make insurance coverage less attractive and thus further depress the proportion of consumers with insurance.

Many states, moreover, regulate the rates and types of policies that can be offered to individuals. Especially in recent years, the regulations have often prevented rates from rising to keep pace with medical expenses and have caused many insurers to incur losses. This

136

situation causes insurers to offer less individual insurance and, in some cases, to abandon the market altogether.

Some states have mandated some form of community rating (for example, New York, California, New Jersey, and Minnesota). New York's law was by far the strictest, requiring essentially pure community rating for all individual and small-group (fewer than fifty employees) insurance. The result has been a major decline in the number of individual and small-group subscribers in a short period. There are conflicting estimates of the magnitude, but even conservative estimates indicate a 16.8 percent decline for individual insurance and 2.6 percent smaller decline for small-group insurance during the fifteen-month period between March 31, 1993, and July 1, 1994 (Institute for Health Policy Solutions 1995, 14–17).

Often the uninsured can fall back on public and private charity medical care and are therefore willing to forgo private insurance. In effect, the uninsured have free insurance from charity. There is political opposition to this free-riding, while there is continuing political support for continuing charity care (Enthoven 1988; 1993, 44; Pauly, Danzon, Feldstein, and Hoff 1991, 8).

The recent growth in the numbers of uninsured consumers is not a symptom of adverse selection and greater competition. At the same time, insurers may be getting better at distinguishing risks. There is a trend toward experience rating for smaller firms over time. This trend may raise problems for guaranteed insurability and oversorting, which are discussed below. Also, better ability to distinguish risks causes rates for some groups to fall and for some to rise. Those for whom rates rise might drop coverage. The workings of insurance markets, especially for individual insurance, are not well understood.

Uninsured versus Insured. Unfortunately, no data allow one to compare health care use for the uninsured versus the insured, with constant relevant demand variables. In particular, the uninsured are much younger, have lower income, and are less likely to work or to work for firms that offer group insurance (Freeman et al. 1987). They also use less medical care, as the adverse selection model predicts, but the difference is surprisingly small.

The employed uninsured use only 49 percent less medical care, according to the 1987 National Medical Care Expenditure Survey (NMCES), conducted by the Department of Health and Human Services. This is not enough difference to suggest large-scale adverse selection. A difference of this magnitude can easily be explained by moral hazard alone. It would be helpful to control for health status in this comparison.

The uninsured's self-reported health status is lower, but they have fewer disability days than the insured (Lefkowitz and Monheit 1991, 9–12; Monheit et al. 1985, 358, 400). A survey conducted by the Robert Wood Johnson Foundation found an even smaller difference in utilization (Freeman et al. 1987, 13).

As another test, one could compare the effect of more complete insurance on utilization for nonexperimental studies (where the data incorporate adverse selection) with that in the RAND experiment, which eliminated selection effects (Manning et al. 1987). This provides evidence that adverse selection is not important. The experimental results are in the low range of the nonexperimental results, but so are the better nonexperimental studies (Manning et al. 1987, 268; Newhouse, Phelps, and Marquis 1980, 383–84).

Selection within Special Programs. A phenomenon that superficially resembles adverse selection has been observed in programs with special rules. Policy makers are sensibly concerned about selection within proposed new programs.

Selection in the federal employee program. Some authors point to cases of apparent adverse selection within the Federal Employees Health Benefits Program (FEHBP) (Price and Mays 1985) or of Medicare beneficiaries into HMOs (Welch 1985). These are both artificial situations because laws and regulations prevent accurate insurance rating that reflects risk and rational management by the groups themselves.

Selection among German sickness funds. Somewhat similar selection is observed among German sickness funds (Finsinger, Kraft, and Pauly 1986). Here, the regulations force the funds to break even and to charge rates that are a fixed percentage of income. About 50 percent of consumers are assigned to a so-called regular sickness fund. About 35 percent of consumers can choose between their assigned regular sickness funds and substitute funds, which must operate on the same financial principles. Those with a choice will select the fund with the most high-income or low-utilization members since such a plan will charge lower taxes or provide better benefits. But the funds will be better off discouraging the lower-income and high-risk consumers from joining.

The regular sickness funds will be left with the lower-income and poorer-health people since many of them are required to participate. Thus, theory suggests that consumers would sort themselves out by income and reduce the ability of the system to redistribute income. This seems borne out empirically (Finsinger, Kraft, and Pauly 1986, 157).

Also, equilibrium can fail to exist. Any new fund that can attract a disproportionately high proportion of high-income workers can undermine any existing fund. Empirically we might expect similar cycling as in the U.S. Federal Employees Program. This does not seem to be happening (Price and Mays 1985, 157).

Proposed special programs. Enthoven has proposed (1980, 1981, 1988, 1993) a plan called the Consumer Choice Health Plan for universal health insurance, mostly provided by competing private HMOs. Enthoven's plan restricts competition and choice in several ways, which have been criticized by William Lynk (1982). Several restrictions are likely to cause selection problems within the program. Most important, he proposed preventing employers from offering only one plan or cross-subsidizing the more complete plans. As we have seen, these are the main tools for group managers to reduce adverse selection within a group. Further, Enthoven would require annual open enrollment by insurers. These restrictions would cause risk-selection problems. Therefore, Enthoven is concerned with selection.

The Dutch government intends to implement a plan similar to and inspired by Enthoven's. Dutch economists are highly concerned with selection problems (van de Ven and van Vliet 1992).

Selection within Private Groups. Pamela Farley and Alan Monheit (1985) have taken the most direct approach to date to see if adverse selection within groups is empirically important. Using a large dataset from the National Medical Care Expenditure Survey, they estimated equations determining the demand for insurance. Actual health care use was included as an explanatory variable. If adverse selection were important, those with high expenditures would have chosen more complete insurance. But Farley and Monheit found evidence of little or no effect. They also found those in groups with many choices had, on average, slightly more complete insurance than those in groups without choices. This is the opposite of what the adverse selection theory would have predicted. These results show that the insurance market has somehow avoided large-scale adverse selection.

The Blue Cross/Blue Shield Argument. Blue Cross/Blue Shield plans often claim that adverse selection is a problem for them and for their customers. This claim betrays a misunderstanding of adverse selection.

Massachusetts Blue Cross/Blue Shield, for example, defines adverse selection as "a significant disparity in risk based on age, sex, and health status between the membership in freedom of choice plans and limited choice/limited access health care plans offered by a single account" (Dailey 1988, 3). This definition differs importantly from the definition used in the economic literature on adverse selection. Age and sex are observable, thus ratable: groups can easily avoid any selection on these bases. Groups may decide not to rate the insurance appropriately for the actual risk, but they can hardly blame the result on adverse selection. Mark Pauly (1985, 651) noted this:

> Indeed, some of the empirical examples of alleged adverse selection in health insurance appear to be caused primarily by Blue Cross' and employer [sic] failure to take profit-maximizing steps to discourage bad risks *who could have been identified* from buying coverage at prices below those appropriate to their expected loss. (emphasis in original)

Further, the management of the Massachusetts Blue Cross/Blue Shield seems to blame selection for group members increasingly dropping out of their 100 percent coverage master medical plan. But this may not be an adverse-selection phenomenon. There is a strong national trend away from such complete coverage. Indeed, Massachusetts is unusual in that so many consumers still have 100 percent traditional coverage.

Blue Cross/Blue Shield of Massachusetts said that rate disparity eventually creates such a large price differential that an account becomes segmented. Lower-risk members choose the HMO, and high-risk members choose the traditional plan. This process looks like the separating equilibrium discussed above. Apparently a group can approximate the Rothschild and Stiglitz adverse-selection result if it ignores risk when setting rates. Is this a bad outcome in some way?

Blue Cross/Blue Shield says yes because the result "undercuts a fundamental principle of health care insurance underwriting, shared or pooled risk" (Dailey 1988, 3). But this statement reveals a common misunderstanding of the nature of insurance.

The Purpose of Insurance. Insurance is designed to pool and shift risk so that each consumer pays a premium roughly equal to his expected loss. Risk-averse consumers will always prefer paying the expected loss to facing the probability of losses. Consumers can always afford insurance, rather than bearing the loss. After all, the insurance will always be cheaper than the loss, unless the loss is almost certain. If the loss is almost certain, there is little need for, nor gain to, insurance. Among people of the same initial risk, insurance redistributes from the lucky to the unlucky. But insurance does not redistribute income between the known low and high risks, or between rich and poor. Redistribution is inconsistent with competition in the insurance market. For a monopolistic insurer, such overpricing and subsidizing would conflict with many ideas of equity or fairness (MacIntyre 1962) and with ideas of honesty and openness of public policy (Pauly 1988a).

Insurance, no matter how competitive or efficient, cannot redistribute income. Efforts to force insurers to redistribute are likely to be undermined by both competition and customer resistance. If observers wish to redistribute income, one simple approach is consistent with efficient insurance markets. The tax system can raise money to subsidize the insurance purchase of the poor or the nonpoor with known high risks. Or tax funds can support public insurance, such as Medicaid and Medicare. (See Pauly, Danzon, Feldstein, and Hoff 1991 for a proposal in this spirit.)

Community Rating. The Massachusetts Blue Cross/Blue Shield writer cited above probably had in mind the idea of community rating, with known high and low risks charged the same premiums. Directly contrary to insurance principles, this idea has been espoused by Blue Cross/Blue Shield plans (MacIntyre 1962), the Kaiser HMOs, and Enthoven (1980, 1981). Community rating requires monopoly power for the insurer. Indeed, Blue Cross and Blue Shield plans used community rating when they had lots of market power, but competition from other insurers forced them to abandon it in the 1950s and 1960s (MacIntyre 1962). Apparently, the Rochester, New York, and Hawaii Blue Cross/ Blue Shield plans are exceptions.

Some—for example, Victor Fuchs—believe that community rating is threatened by the new competitiveness of U.S. health care (1986, 252–54). This view is wrong, largely for two reasons. First, as discussed, community rating has been rare for decades. Second, the new competitiveness is primarily a development in the health care market, not in the health insurance market.

By now, community rating is rare, except in some HMOs, particularly the Kaiser HMOs. Kaiser, with a large head start, has created a valuable brand name, probably the most valuable brand name in health care. Federal HMO regulation, which formerly required federally qualified HMOs to community rate, has protected Kaiser from competition from experience-rated HMOs. Thus, Kaiser has had enough market power to use community rating. In the 1980s, increasing competition from new experience-rated HMOs and PPOs is decreasing Kaiser's market power. And the federal HMO law has been amended to allow experience rating. Responding to the resulting increase in competition, in 1989 Kaiser adopted more accurate rating for some of its larger clients, based on age and sex. This is a retreat from community rating, though Kaiser calls the rating plan adjusted community rating (Mullen 1989).

Regardless, community rating is inefficient. It prices the insurance too high for low risks and too low for high risks. Thus, it leads the high risks to purchase too much insurance and leads the low risks to purchase too little, or perhaps to do without it altogether. In this respect, community rating is worse than the separating equilibrium under adverse selection (Pauly 1970; 1988b, 52; Crocker and Snow 1986). Community rating exacerbates adverse selection. Insurers forced to lose money on high-risk consumers are less likely to encourage them to enroll. Finally, MacIntyre (1962) argued that community rating is inequitable. It forces low-risk consumers, many of whom are poor, to subsidize high-risk consumers whether they are poor or wealthy. Huang and Rosett (1972) found that community rating in Rochester indeed redistributed income from the poor to the wealthy.

An employer's refusal to rate insurance policies by age can be viewed as community rating within its group. This policy has one particularly bad effect. Young workers are overcharged so much that they often refuse to buy insurance, even when it is subsidized by the employer. Indeed, this is probably the main reason the employed uninsured are relatively young. Employers have traditionally ignored age in pricing insurance. Until recently, health insurance was such a small part of labor costs that employers could disregard the inefficiency caused by purposely ignoring age in rating the policies. In the future, as health insurance grows as a share of compensation, I would expect to see more age rating within groups, with compensating changes in the age-wage profile.

What Are the Real Problems?

Adverse selection of health insurance is apparently not a major problem. If so, why has so much ink been spilled about it? There are and have been real problems in insurance markets. They are the results not of adverse selection but rather of some related phenomena.

Guaranteed Insurability. Consumers are concerned that they might become a high risk at some time. If this were to happen and the consumer were simultaneously to lose his insurance, obtaining new insurance would be expensive. Coverage against this risk is called guaranteed insurability.

This chance of becoming a high risk is covered by most health insurance policies. First, group policies usually include provisions for conversion to individual (nongroup) coverage if membership in the group is terminated. Second, individual insurance itself usually contains clauses so that neither can it be canceled nor can the rates be changed for specific individuals regardless of their health status or health expenditures.

A small change in the types of policies since the mid-1970s demonstrates one ill effect of state insurance regulation. As early as 1968, "guaranteed renewable" policies were described as probably the most common (Reed and Carr 1970, 82). By the mid-1970s, most individual insurance was of this type. Guaranteed renewable policies meant that the insurer could not cancel the policy under any circumstances. Further, rates could not be raised for an individual no matter what the loss experience. Rates could be raised only for a whole class of customers within a state. Since then, as mentioned, in many states insurance regulators have not allowed individual insurance rates to rise to keep pace with rising costs. As a result, many insurers have dropped out of the individual insurance market, and those remaining have largely shifted to a type of insurance that is slightly less secure for the consumers. Both changes have contributed to the increase in the uninsured.

The new form of insurance now dominant is called optionally renewable. With this type of policy, insurers still cannot cancel or raise rates for an individual, no matter how high the expenses. Rates can be raised only for a whole class of business within a state. The insurer however, can choose to withdraw from insuring a class in a state. Most insurers still writing individual insurance are major companies with little risk of withdrawing, but still the risk to the consumer is higher than before (Raymond 1992). Some consumers could simultaneously lose their insurance and become high risks. Because of state regulation, this risk has become a bit worse.

Individual insurance is important for covering those without access to group coverage. And individual insurance is regulated in ways that discourage it. For some reason, individual insurance has not received much research or policy attention. More research on individual insurance is greatly needed.

Community rating has one advantage. When combined with open enrollment, community rating provides insurance against the risk of simultaneously losing insurance and becoming a high risk. But since it requires much insurer market power, this combination has long disappeared from most of the market. A vestige remains where Blue Cross/ Blue Shield plans offer open enrollment. It is vestigial because community rating is limited to individual members or even to the high-risk individuals who joined through open enrollment. Thus, the rates are high. Also, the insurance for those who use open enrollment is generally less complete (U.S. General Accounting Office 1986, 15–19).

Job switching. When individuals switch jobs, they can run a risk of losing their insurance. Clearly, this risk is greater if the new employer offers no insurance or offers insurance that excludes preexisting conditions. Some observers believe that this problem is growing. As a result, some individuals may stay in less-favored jobs when another job would be better for them and more efficient for the economy. Research has shown that this job-lock effect of group health insurance is noticeable, though not huge. Using data from the 1987 National Medical Expenditure Survey, Brigitte Madrian estimated that job-lock reduces the voluntary turnover rate of those with employer-provided group health insurance from 16 to 12 percent per year (1993).

The Elderly and Medicare. Before the Medicare programs took effect in 1966, many insurance policies ended at the retirement age of sixty-five. By that age, some people had become high risks. Some lost their group insurance coverage. The theory of adverse selection predicts that the high risks would buy the optimal level of insurance coverage at appropriately high rates and the low risks would buy less coverage or even none at all.

In fact, the elderly were less likely to buy health insurance. A pre-Medicare survey taken in 1956 found that 63 percent of those aged from forty-five to fifty-four had health insurance, while only 31 percent of those over 65 did (Akerlof 1970, 492). Nongroup insurance is far more costly; one would expect that fewer retired people would buy insurance than would working people.

Observers believed that some of those uninsured older than sixty-five were high risks who relied on family assistance, charity, or welfare rather than pay the high insurance rates appropriate to their expected costs. Voters did not like to contemplate these high-risk older people being in this predicament. Also, some uninsured elderly were free-riding on charity provided by others, which seemed both unfair and inefficient. Consumers might have been willing to insure against risk if there were a perfect and costless insurance market. These judgments formed part of the basis for the political support for Medicare.

The problem of some high-risk elderly without insurance has been attributed to adverse selection (Akerlof 1970, 492; Fuchs 1986, 311). That direction implies the market failed to exist for high-risk elderly consumers—a claim for which no evidence has been offered. It is far more likely that the implicit insurance, provided by family and public or private charity, was simply more attractive than regular insurance for many high-risk elderly.

Costly Sorting. The work of Mark Pauly (1970) and Keith Crocker and

Arthur Snow (1986) shows that if sorting consumers by risk is costless, it always improves economic efficiency to sort more accurately. In other words, sharper differentiation of risks using readily available information such as age, sex, location, or occupation always improves efficiency.

This strong result disappears when one considers that sorting and information gathering are costly. The sorting devices used in health insurance include medical records review, medical examination, and testing; a controversial example is testing for the AIDS virus. Profitable self-selection can be induced by an otherwise inefficient plan design or marketing. Well-baby and maternity care, for example, can be included without coinsurance or deductible to attract families with healthy children. Coverage for these services was expanded by California and Oregon Blue Cross and Blue Shield plans to counter favorable selection by HMOs (Goldberg and Greenberg 1977a, 77, 98). HMO offices can be strategically located in neighborhoods with low health care utilization.

When sorting is costly, there is an optimal amount of sorting. Further, the market will do too much sorting—simply because the low risks always benefit from better sorting, as their rates go down. The insurer of the low risks might be better off with more information. But the high risks are hurt because they face higher rates when their risk level is revealed to insurers. Sorting provides some efficiency gains but also transfers wealth from the high risks to the low risks and to the low risks' insurer. Therefore, the low risks and the insurer will cooperate in improving information beyond the point where it is socially optimal or efficient (Borenstein 1989).

Managers use several strategies to reduce wasteful oversorting within groups. They invariably limit the number of health insurers at any one time, limit the information the insurers can have about members, and limit or prohibit insurers from choosing among group members. Partly for these reasons, group insurance is cheaper than individual insurance. Outside of groups, insurers expend too much effort sorting consumers by risk. Further, the expense of costly sorting no doubt discourages the purchase of insurance in the individual market and contributes to the problem of the uninsured.

Adverse Selection, Overinsurance, and Managed Care

We have seen that adverse selection is apparently a minor phenomenon. The theoretical analysis shows that one of its effects is to cause some consumers to have less complete insurance. As discussed, there are powerful tax, regulatory, and historical forces pushing the equilibrium in the direction of overinsurance. If adverse selection partially offsets these forces, it makes the equilibrium extent of insurance closer to the optimum.

Roger Feldman and Bryan Dowd (1991) have shown that adverse selection is likely to reinforce incentives for plans to manage care aggressively, for example, by utilization review. Since some incentives already lead to too little and too passive managed care just as for overinsurance, adverse selection pushes the equilibrium closer to the optimum in this dimension. Especially within groups with scant wasteful oversorting, a little adverse selection may be a good thing.

In sum, there is probably much less adverse selection in health insurance and health care markets than the policy debate would suggest. Government policies designed to limit adverse selection by restrictions on consumer choice probably represent an overreaction. But the related problems of guaranteed insurability and oversorting in individual insurance markets are worthy of more attention.

8
Conclusion

There has always been more competition in medical care than meets the eye, though there has always been monopoly as well. Empirical research has firmly rejected both the theories of perfect monopoly and perfect competition. Recent developments on several fronts have led to the market rapidly becoming more competitive.

Competition Has Been Increasing

The American Medical Association and the state and local societies have lost their control of hospital privileges, thus much of their power to reduce competition among physicians. This has occurred mostly because of a few key antitrust decisions. The AMA has lost political influence as well, as shown by its inability to stop either Medicare in 1966 or the expansion in medical schools in the 1960s and 1970s. The new physicians have more incentive to compete aggressively.

In terms of competition and efficiency, health insurance got off to a bad start by following the Blue Cross/Blue Shield plans, with their 100 percent, hands-off coverage. But, in recent years, positive changes have occurred. Consumer copayment, mostly as coinsurance and deductibles, has soared. Besides reducing demand through reducing moral hazard, higher copayments encourage consumer search and choice of low-cost providers. Health maintenance organizations, with their physician contracts and utilization controls, have grown rapidly. Perhaps most important, preferred provider organizations have flourished. PPOs directly encourage discounting by contract and improve consumer information; they also use administrative utilization controls. Further, much of traditional insurance has adopted utilization controls.

Medicare, conversely, has been steadily becoming more anticompetitive. Medicare's original benefit design had significant cost controls in the physician deductible, coinsurance, and balance billing. Medigap supplementary insurance has eroded the cost controls to the point that many Medicare beneficiaries' insurance has 100 percent coverage for physicians and hospitals. In the past few years, there have been two major policy changes in Medicare. One is helpful, the other probably not.

Medicare's introduction of the prospective payment system for hospitals partially emulates a competitive market and seems to be improving efficiency and reducing costs. PPS can be viewed as a form of price regulation or as a more efficient and more procompetitive way for the government to purchase services. Some private insurers are using a similar system. In contrast, physician reimbursement policy is becoming less favorable to competition. The movement toward the resource-based relative value scale and especially the severe restrictions on balance billing are likely to reduce competition, efficiency, and consumer access.

Recent National Health Care Plans and Medicare Reforms

In 1994, the Clinton administration proposed a comprehensive national health plan, its Health Security Act. Though the proposal started with wide support, it died without coming to a vote. Despite rhetorical bows to competition, the proposal was actually quite destructive of competition. Monopolistic regional alliances were created with great power over health insurerers. Perhaps the most serious was the imposition of binding price controls on health insurers and, even more seriously, on physicians and hospitals.

As a result, the proposal was widely attacked as being more regulatory, centralized, and anticompetitive than necessary. The proposal died partly because of this criticism (Bowman 1995). The critiques came from economists, including an open letter from 565 economists organized by John Lott (Enthoven 1993b; Feldstein and Feldstein 1993; Lott 1994). Not surprisingly, congressional Republicans were also among the critics (Rogers 1994; Rogers and Stout 1994).

Ironically, the Republicans' Medicare Preservation Act of 1995, a proposal for reforming Medicare, includes the same key idea. It is based on reducing the growth of Medicare spending by imposing tight price controls on hospitals and physicians (Kinsley 1995; Kendall 1995). The Republican Congress has appropriated the Clinton administration's most anticompetitive idea as the centerpiece of its plan. As we have seen, the likely result is large hidden costs imposed on the Medicare enrollees. Perhaps the Republicans intend to drive both Medicare enrollees and their physicians out of fee-for-service medicine by making conditions intolerable. But this is needlessly harmful to competition, innovation, and efficiency in health care, just as the Clinton plan was. In some minor ways, the Republican proposal is less harmful to competition than the Clinton plan (Goodman 1995). But the central fact is that the 1994–1996 Republican Congress has adopted price controls, not competition, as the key to Medicare reform.

Is More Competition Better?

Full coverage of this topic would lead us far beyond the scope of this book. Most observers, particularly economists, favor more competition in most parts of the health care industy. The courts and antitrust enforcement agencies have generally endorsed competion. But the changes introduced by increasing competition are not universally popular.

Increasing competition has reduced the ability of hospitals and physicians to cross-subsidize the poor. There has long been an implicit bargain between the government and health care providers and, to a lesser extent, insurers. In return for not disturbing their market power, the providers supply some free or subsidized care. For some insurers, the implicit quid pro quo was provision of some individual coverage on an open-enrollment basis.

In effect, consumers pay a hidden tax administered by monopolistic providers and insurers. Some proceeds of the tax are used to subsidize care for the poor. More competition will reduce the monopoly rents of the providers and insurers and presumably reduce cross-subsidization.

Victor Fuchs (1986, 352–54), Mark Schlesinger (1987), and Arnold Relman (1992) raised the possibility that less cross-subsidization may be a bad thing: the poor may end up with smaller total transfers. Relman believed that competition leads to less ethical behavior by physicians by making poor ethics more profitable.

There is surprisingly little evidence available on any of these issues. Richard Frank and David Salkever (1991) found that where more hospitals are competing in a local market, more charity care is provided, not less. But Mark Schlesinger, Judy Bentkover, David Blumenthal, Robert Musacchio, and Janet Miller (1987) reported that physicians generally perceived better access to care for the poor in more concentrated hospital markets.

On the issue of health care for the poor, Mark Pauly (1988a) favored replacing the current hidden tax and subsidy system with an explicit one. He believed that it would be more efficient and more consistent with democratic government. Consumers and voters could easily see the tax and subsidy. The system would be, as the Germans say, more transparent.[1]

---

1. German discussions of public policy offer wide agreement on the goal of

Fuchs (1986, 347, 348) also raised the cross-subsidy issue for medical research and education. In the past, payments for hospital care have gone to support such activites. Increasing competition reduces the monopoly rents available for such cross-subsidies.

As discussed, hospital competition occurs partly on nonprice or quality dimensions. Many believe that medical care quality, at least in the sense of costly, high-tech procedures and equipment, is already too high. If so, more hospital competition might make matters worse and raise costs and prices without commensurate increases in consumer benefit. Research with the latest data suggests that hospital competition now focuses more on price. The fear that more competition would raise cost and price has subsided (Zwansiger and Melnick 1988).

Some observers now have the opposite concern. David Dranove and Mark Satterthwaite (1990) showed theoretically that more competition can lead to quality that is too low if competition improves price information more than quality information. As they noted, this unfortunate outcome is more likely if quality is already lower than optimal. James Robinson (1988) argued along a similar line that new developments in the economic theory of signaling make it unclear that more competition will be good. Wyszewianski, Wheeler, and Donabedian (1982) believed current quality is too low and suggested that steps be taken to keep competition from driving it lower.

Other observers, such as Mancur Olson (1985), believed the opposite: current quality is typically higher than optimal. The effect of competition (and regulation) on quality and other nonprice aspects of care deserves continuing research.

At times directly competing physicians should cooperate for the patient's benefit. The most obvious case occurs when a patient switches physicians in the middle of treatment. At the least, the newly selected physician should obtain the patient's medical records from his direct competitor. Often he needs to discuss the case with the physician. Fuchs (1986, 352) raised a concern that this free exchange of information may be hampered by sharper competition among physicians.

There is a problem here. As competition improves both price and quality information, patients are likely to switch physicians more often, and the switches are likely to be more systematic (less random). Some physicians could harm their rivals by withholding information with little danger of retaliation. Legally, medical records are the pa-

---

transparency, meaning that voters can see what is happening. I would favor importing that goal into U.S. policy decisions. One immediate implication is that the hidden cross-subsidies in the U.S. health system should be eliminated in favor of explicit taxes and subsidies.

tient's property. But the formal medical records do not contain all useful information.

Another example of the need for cooperation among competitors is the problem of coverage for emergencies, especially for specialists. Physicians must arrange for coverage of their specialty. Typically, the other specialists who provide the coverage are direct competitors. Usually, the covering physician transfers the patient back after the emergency. Again, there is a tension between cooperation and competition.

Even if one prefers more competition, it is no panacea. At best, competition can reduce the cost of medical care, improve efficiency, and allow for greater consumer choice. But more competition cannot provide medical care for poor people or support high levels of medical research. These activities require charitable or governmental action, a requirement made more obvious as competition reduces the monopoly rents used to cross-subsidize these activities in the past. Further, competition and government involvement are not mutually exclusive. Competition advocate Alain Enthoven (1978, 1980, 1987, 1993), for example, favored extensive government regulation of the ground rules for competition. On a broader scale, antitrust enforcement also can be viewed as governmental regulation of the ground rules for competition.

Competition Can Be Encouraged

The most important procompetitive reform would be tax reform to limit or end the tax deductibility of private health insurance. The least disruptive approach is to cap the employer's deductions at a dollar amount sufficient to cover minimal basic insurance with high cost sharing and perhaps managed care as well. Requiring that most insurance be bought with after-tax dollars would further discourage the overly complete, hands-off insurance that most harms competition.

Next, consumer cost sharing should be increased in the traditional fee-for-service parts of the Medicare and Medicaid programs. In Medicaid, a distinction needs to be made between the poorest consumers, for whom 100 percent coverage might be best, and the rest, for whom modest cost sharing would be useful. It should be made easier for Medicare and Medicaid members to enroll in private HMOs and PPOs. This enrollment would allow the government to take advantage of the competing private sector's ability to control costs while respecting consumer choice. But experience with the small Medicare HMO program and Medicaid experiments shows that this reform poses difficult political challenges.

Last, the growing application of antitrust law to health care should be continued. In recent years, the U.S. Department of Justice, the Federal Trade Commission, and the state attorneys general have increased their enforcement activity in health care. This has borne generally good results.[2] Indeed, Clark Havighurst (1995, 2–3) calls health care antitrust "one of the great victories in the history of antitrust law."

Finally, anticompetitive regulations at the state level still hinder competition in both health care and health insurance markets. Examples include restrictive licensure laws, mandated benefits, rules limiting HMO policies, rules against PPOs, and certificate-of-need laws that hinder hospital competition. In many states, these laws are being repealed. This trend should continue.

Research on Competition

The tremendous public policy interest in improving competition and efficiency in health care leads directly to a demand for continued research. We need a better idea of what enhances and what harms competition. The health care industry is changing so fast and is so poorly understood that there is a need for continuing research of a purely descriptive kind.

Also, scientific interest in the economics of imperfect competition is growing. Since the health care industry is rich in examples of imperfect competition from monopolistic competition to professional collusion, the industry attracts research. Thus, some research on health care competition results from scientific curiosity.

Since the basic causal mechanisms of competition are sometimes obscure and even counterintuitive, both empirical and theoretical analyses are necessary. Imperfect competition is often closely tied to the specific history of specific competitors. General results of the kind found in the theory of perfect competition will be rare. There will always be a demand for empirical and historical studies of specific local markets at specific times.

The Future of Health Care Competition

Private insurers, HMOs, and PPOs are experimenting and innovating. Old legal and professional barriers to competition are tumbling down. Even without new procompetitive policies, the trends are leading to a more competitive and efficient health care system. The health care sys-

---

2. Antitrust controversies, of course, continue. Of particular interest is one concerning physician networks and their ability to negotiate with HMOs and PPOs (Havighurst 1995).

tem is also becoming more humane because it is responding more to consumer values and choices. Still, more competition does not mean perfect competition. And even perfect competition could not solve all policy problems in health care.

There are political pressures for policies that would slow the positive changes we observe. Some states are already enacting anticompetitive regulations. But the biggest threat to future competition in health care is probably from certain types of national health insurance or national health care reform systems that restrict competition, innovation, and flexibility, for example, by instituting price controls and limiting choice of health plan. A national health insurance system and similar policy changes are not necessarily harmful to competition. They could be designed to encourage competition, for example, by limiting the tax-deductibility of health insurance premiums. Federal and state governments will probably avoid the most restrictive policies; health care competition and efficiency should continue to improve.

References

Aaron, Henry J., and William B. Schwartz. *The Painful Prescription: Rationing Hospital Care.* Washington, D.C.: Brookings Institution, 1984.

Acton, Jan Paul. "Nonmonetary Factors in the Demand for Medical Services: Some Empirical Evidence." *Journal of Political Economy* 83, no. 3 (June 1975): 595–614.

Adamache, Killard W., and Frank A. Sloan. "Competition between Non-Profit and For-Profit Health Insurers." *Journal of Health Economics* 2 (1983): 225–43.

Agreement between American Hospital Association and the Blue Cross Plans. Chicago, March 1, 1954.

Agreement Relating to the Collective Service Mark "Blue Shield." Chicago, 1951.

Akerloff, George A. "The Market for Lemons: Quality Uncertainty and the Market Mechanism." *Quarterly Journal of Economics* 84, no. 3 (August 1970): 488–500.

Alchian, Armen A. *Some Economics of Property.* Santa Monica, Calif.: RAND Corp., May 1961.

Alchian, Armen A., and Harold Demsetz. "Production, Information Costs and Economic Organization." *American Economic Review* 62, no. 5 (December 1972): 777–95.

Alchian, Armen A., and Ruben Kessel. "Competition, Monopoly, and the Pursuit of Money." In *Aspects of Labor Economics*, National Bureau of Economic Research, Special Conference Series, vol. 14, pp. 157–75. Princeton: Princeton University Press, 1962.

American Hospital Association. *Approval Program for Blue Cross Plans.* Chicago: AHA, 1964.

American Hospital Association Board of Trustees. *Service Benefits or Cash Indemnity in Hospital Prepayment.* Chicago: American Hospital Association, 1960.

American Medical Association v. United States, 317 U.S. 519 (1943).

American Medical International and Amisub (French Hospital): Final Order and Opinion. Docket No. 9158, Federal Trade Commission, July 2, 1984.

Andersen, Ronald, and Odin W. Anderson. *A Decade of Health Services.*

Chicago: University of Chicago Press, 1970.

Anderson, Keith B. "Regulation, Market Structure and Hospital Costs: Comment." *Southern Economic Journal* 58, no. 2 (Oct. 1991): 528–34.

Anderson, Odin W. *Blue Cross since 1929: Accountability and the Public Trust.* Cambridge: Ballinger, 1975.

Arnould, Richard J., and Lawrence M. DeBrock. "The Effect of Provider Control of Blue Shield Plans on Health Care Markets." *Economic Inquiry* 23, no. 3 (July 1985): 449–76.

Arnould, Richard J., and David Eisenstadt. "The Effects of Provider-controlled Blue Shield Plans: Regulatory Options." In *A New Approach to the Economics of Health Care,* edited by Mancur Olson. pp. 337–58. Washington, D.C.: American Enterprise Institute, 1981.

Auster, Richard D., and Ronald L. Oaxaca. "Identification of Supplier Induced Demand in the Health Care Sector." *Journal of Human Resources* 16, no. 3 (summer 1981): 327–42.

Baker, Jonathan B. "The Antitrust Analysis of Hospital Mergers and the Transformation of the Hospital Industry." *Law and Contemporary Problems* 51, no. 2 (spring 1988).

———. "Vertical Restraints among Hospitals, Physicians and Health Insurers that Raise Rivals' Costs." *American Journal of Law and Medicine* 14, nos. 2–3 (1989): 147–69.

Barton, David M. "Alternative Institutional Arrangements for Medical Care Insurance." Ph.D. diss., University of Virginia, 1974.

Bays, Carson W. "Why Most Private Hospitals Are Nonprofit." *Journal of Policy Analysis and Management* 2, no. 3 (spring 1983): 366–85.

———. "Specification Error in the Estimation of Hospital Cost Functions." *Review of Economics and Statistics* 62, no. 2 (May 1980): 302–5.

Beazoglou, Tryfon, Dennis Heffley, and Subhash Ray. "Provider Entry in a Bounded Market: An Alternative View of 'Induced Demand' for Health Services." University of Connecticut, November 1986.

Becker, Edmund R., and Frank A. Sloan. "Hospital Ownership and Performance." *Economic Inquiry* 23, no. 1 (January 1985): 21–36.

Becker, Gary. *The Economics of Discrimination.* 2d ed. Chicago: University of Chicago Press, 1971.

Begun, James W., and Roger Feldman. "Policy and Research on Health Manpower Regulations: Never Too Late to Deregulate." *Advances in Health Economics and Health Services Research* 11 (1990): 79–110.

Benham, Lee. "The Effect of Advertising on the Price of Eyeglasses." *Journal of Law and Economics* 25, no. 2 (October 1972): 337–52.

———. "Guilds and the Form of Competition in the Health Care Sector." In *Competition in the Health Care Sector: Past, Present, and Future,* Proceedings of a conference sponsored by the Bureau of Economics, Federal Trade Commission, March 1978, edited by Warren Greenberg, pp. 363–74. Germantown, Md.: Aspen, 1978.

Benham, Lee, and Alexandra Benham. "Regulating through the Professions: A Perspective on Information Control." *Journal of Law and Economics* 18, no. 2 (October 1975): 421–48.

Benham, Lee, Alexander Maurizi, and Melvin W. Reder. "Migration, Location and Remuneration of Medical Personnel: Physicians and Dentists." *Review of Economics and Statistics* 50 (August 1968): 332–47.

Benjamini, Yael, and Yoav Benjamini. "The Choice among Medical Insurance Plans." *American Economic Review* 76, no. 1 (March 1986): 221–27.

Berlant, Jeffrey L. *Profession and Monopoly: A Study of Medicine in the United States and Great Britain.* Berkeley: University of California Press, 1975.

————. "The Sociology of a Benevolent Cartel." Presented at the Program on Antitrust in the Health Care Field, National Health Lawyers Association, Washington, D.C., January 7–8, 1981.

Berman, Howard. "Comment: Competition among Health Insurers." In *Competition in the Health Care Sector: Past, Present, and Future,* Proceedings of a conference sponsored by the Bureau of Economics, Federal Trade Commission, March 1978, edited by Warren Greenberg, pp. 189–206. Germantown, Md.: Aspen, 1978.

Blackstone, Erwin A., and Joseph P. Fuhr, Jr. "Hospital Mergers and Antitrust: An Economic Analysis." *Journal of Health Politics, Policy and Law* 14, no. 2 (summer 1989): 383–403.

Blair, Roger D., Paul B. Ginsburg, and Ronald J. Vogel. "Blue Cross-Blue Shield Administration Costs: A Study of Nonprofit Health Insurers." *Economic Inquiry* 13, no. 2 (July 1975): 237–51.

Blue Cross and Blue Shield Association v. Community Mutual Insurance Company and State of Ohio, Settlement Agreement, U.S. District Court for the Northern District of Ohio, Case No. C85-7872, May 20, 1987.

Blue Cross Association. *Membership Standards of Blue Cross Association.* Chicago: BCA, November 21, 1981.

Blue Cross and Blue Shield of Massachusetts. "In the Matter of Proposed Agreement between Blue Cross of Massachusetts, Inc. and Medical West Community Health Plan, Inc. Exclusive Provider Agreement," Response to Notice of Public Hearing, Rate Setting Commission, Division of Insurance (November 23, 1988).

Blue Cross Plan Approval Program of the American Hospital Association. Chicago: American Hospital Association, September 1946.

Blumberg, Mark S. "Medical Society Regulation of Fees in Boston, 1780–1820. *Journal of the History of Medicine and Allied Sciences* 39, no. 3 (July 1984): 303–38.

Bond, Ronald S., John E. Kwoka, Jr., John J. Phelan, and Ira Taylor Whitten. *Effects of Restrictions on Advertising and Commercial Practice in the Professions: The Case of Optometry.* Staff report, Bureau of Economics,

Federal Trade Commission. Washington, D.C.: FTC, 1980.

Booth, Alan, and Nicholas Babchuk. "Seeking Health Care from New Resources." *Journal of Health and Social Behavior* 13, no. 1 (March 1972): 90–99.

Borenstein, Severin. "The Economics of Costly Risk Sorting in Competitive Insurance Markets." *International Review of Law and Economics* 9, no. 1 (June 1989): 25–39.

Borjas, George J., H. E. Frech III, and Paul B. Ginsburg. "Property Rights and Wages: The Case of Nursing Homes." *Journal of Human Resources* 17, no. 2 (spring 1983): 231–46.

Bowman, Karlyn H. "Learning from the Imperfect Debate." *Health Affairs* 14, no. 1 (September 1995): 27–30.

Bunker, John P., and Bryon Wm. Brown, Jr. "The Physician-Patient as an Informed Consumer of Surgical Services." *New England Journal of Medicine* 290, no. 19 (May 9, 1974): 1051–55.

Butz, David A. "Durable Good Monopoly and Best-Price Provisions." *American Economic Review* 80, no. 5 (December 1990): 1062–76.

Cain, Glen. "The Economic Analysis of Labor Market Discrimination." In *Handbook of Labor Economics*, edited by Orley Ashenfelter and Richard Layard, chap. 13, pp. 693–786. Amsterdam: North-Holland, 1986.

Carlton, Dennis W., and Jeffrey M. Perloff. *Modern Industrial Organization*. Glenview, Ill.: Scott, Foresman/Little Brown, 1990.

Carr, John W., and Paul J. Feldstein. "The Relationship of Cost to Hospital Size." *Inquiry* 4, no. 2 (summer 1967): 355–66.

Cave, Jonathan A. K. "Subsidy Equilibrium and Multi-Option Insurance Markets." *Advances in Health Economics and Health Services Research* 6 (1985): 27–46.

California Dental Service. *CDS Newsletter*. July–August 1981.

———. *CDS Newsletter*. September–October 1983.

Clark, Robert Charles. "Does the Nonprofit Form Fit the Hospital Industry?" *Harvard Law Review* 93, no. 7 (May 1980): 1416–89.

Cohen, Harold. "Variations in Costs among Hospitals of Different Sizes." *Southern Economic Journal* 33, no. 3 (June 1967): 45–65.

Comanor, William S. *National Health Insurance in Ontario: The Effects of a Policy of Cost Control*. Washington, D.C.: American Enterprise Institute, 1980.

Comanor, William S., and H. E. Frech III. "Vertical Agreements: Reply." *American Economic Review* 77, no. 5 (December 1987): 1069–72.

Cook, Paul W., Jr. "Fact and Fancy on Identical Bids." *Harvard Business Review* 41, no. 1 (January–February 1963): 67–72.

Cowing, T. G., A. G. Holtman, and S. Powers. "Hospital Cost Analysis:

A Survey and Evaluation of Recent Studies." *Advances in Health Economics and Health Services Research* 4 (1983): 257–303.

Crocker, Keith J., and Arthur Snow. "The Efficiency Effects of Categorical Discrimination in the Insurance Industry." *Journal of Political Economy* 94, no. 2 (April 1986): 321–44.

Cromwell, Jerry, and Janet B. Mitchell. "Physician-induced Demand for Surgery." *Journal of Health Economics* 5, no. 4 (December 1986): 293–313.

Culyer, Anthony J., Alan Maynard, and Alan Williams. "Alternative Systems of Health Care Provision: An Essay on Motes and Beams." In *A New Approach to the Economics of Health Care,* edited by Mancur Olson, pp. 131–50. Washington, D.C.: American Enterprise Institute, 1981.

Custer, William S. "Hospital Attributes and Physician Prices." *Southern Economic Journal* 52, no. 4 (April 1986): 1010–27.

Danzon, Patricia M. "The Hidden Costs of Budget-constrained Health Insurance Systems." In *Health Policy Reform,* edited by Robert Helms, pp. 256–92. Washington, D.C.: AEI Press, 1993.

Dailey, Edward J. (general counsel, Blue Cross/Blue Shield). "Letter to Nancy Turnbull (deputy commissioner of insurance) re Regulatory Submission of Exclusive Provider Arrangement." October 11, 1988.

Delaware Health Council. *Health Plan for Delaware.* Wilmington, Delaware: Delaware Health Council, Inc. and Statewide Health Coordinating Council, Bureau of Health Planning and Resources Development, 1984.

De Vany, Arthur S., Donald R. House, and Thomas R. Saving. "The Role of Patient Time in the Pricing of Dental Services: The Fee-Provider Density Relation Explained." *Southern Economic Journal* 49, no. 3 (January 1983): 669–80.

Donahue, John H. III, and James Heckman. "Continuous versus Episodic Change: The Impact of Civil Rights Policy on the Economic Status of Blacks." *Journal of Economic Literature* 39, no. 4 (December 1991): 1603–43.

Dorfman, Robert, and Peter Steiner. "Optimal Advertising and Optimal Quality." *American Economic Review* 44, no. 6 (December 1954): 826–36.

Dowd, Bryan, Roger Feldman, Steven Cassou, and Michael Fince. "Health Plan Choice and the Utilization of Health Care Services." *Review of Economics and Statistics* 123, no. 1 (February 1991): 85–93.

Dranove, David. "Demand Inducement and the Physician-Patient Relationship." *Economic Inquiry* 26, no. 2 (April 1980): 281–98.

Dranove, David, and Mark A. Satterthwaite. "Monopolistic Competition When Price and Quality Are Not Perfectly Observable." University of Chicago School of Business, March 27, 1990.

159

————. "The Implications for Resource-based Relative Value Scales for Physicians' Fees, Incomes and Specialty Choices." In *Regulating Doctors' Fees: Competition, Benefits and Controls under Medicare*, edited by H. E. Frech III, pp. 52–70. Washington, D.C.: AEI Press, 1991.

Dranove, David, Mark Satterthwaite, and Jody Sindelar. "The 'New Competitiveness' in Health Care: Some Implications for Price and Quantity." *Inquiry* 23, no. 4 (winter 1986): 429–31.

Dranove, David, and Mark Shanley. "A Note on the Relational Aspects of Hospital Market Definitions." *Journal of Health Economics* 8, no. 4 (February 1990): 473–78.

Dranove, David, Mark Shanley, and Carol Simon. "Is Hospital Competition Wasteful? No!" University of Chicago, July 12, 1991.

Dranove, David, Mark Shanley, and William White. "Hospital Pricing Behavior under Competition." University of Chicago, February 1991.

Dranove, David, and William D. White. "Changes in Hospital Market Share at the DRG Level." University of Chicago, March 5, 1990.

Dyckman, Zachary. *Physicians: A Study of Physicians' Fees*. Staff report, Council of Wage and Price Stability. Washington, D.C.: U.S. Government Printing Office, March 1978.

Eisenberg, Barry S. "Information Exchange among Competitors: The Issue of Relative Value Scales for Physicians' Services." *Journal of Law and Economics* 23, no. 2 (October 1980): 441–60.

Eisenstadt, David M. "Health Care Antitrust Analysis: Thinking Through the Issues." Presented at Trends in Antitrust Healthcare Conference, American Bar Association (October 1990).

Eisenstadt, David M., and Thomas E. Kennedy. "Control and Behavior of Nonprofit Firms: The Case of Blue Shield." *Southern Economic Journal* 48, no. 1 (July 1981): 26–36.

Enterline, Philip E., J. Corbett McDonald, Alison D. McDonald, Lise Davigu, and Vera Salter. "Effects of 'Free' Medical Care on Medical Practice—The Quebec Experience." *New England Journal of Medicine* 288, no. 22 (May 31, 1973): 1152–55.

Enterline, Philip E., J. Corbett McDonald, Alison D. McDonald, and Vivian Henderson. "Physician's Working Hours and Patients Seen before and after National Health Insurance: 'Free' Medical Care and Medical Practice." *Medical Care* 13, no. 2 (February 1975): 95–103.

Enthoven, Alain C. "Competition of Alternative Delivery Systems." In *Competition in the Health Care Sector: Past, Present, and Future*, Proceeding of a conference sponsored by the Bureau of Economics, Federal Trade Commission, March 1978, edited by Warren Greenberg, pp. 255–78. Germantown, Md.: Aspen, 1978.

————. "Supply-Side Economics of Health Care and Consumer Choice Health Plan." In *A New Approach to the Economics of Health Care*, edited by Mancur Olson, pp. 465–90. Washington, D.C.: American Enterprise Institute, 1981.

————. *Health Plan: The Only Practical Solution to the Soaring Cost of Medical Care.* Reading, Mass.: Addison-Wesley, 1980.

————. "The U.S. Health Care Economy: From Guild to Market in Ten Years." *Health Policy* 7, no. 2 (1987): 241–51.

————. "Managed Competition: An Agenda for Action." *Health Affairs* 7, no. 3 (summer 1988): 26–47.

————. "The History and Principles of Managed Competition." *Health Affairs* 12 supp. (1993a): 24–48.

————. "A Good Health Care Idea Gone Bad." *Wall Street Journal* (October 7, 1993b).

Evans, Robert C. "Behavioral Cost Functions for Hospitals." *Canadian Journal of Economics* 4, no. 2 (1971): 198–215.

————. "Supplier-induced Demand: Some Empirical Evidence and Implications." In *The Economics of Health and Medical Care: Proceedings of a Conference Held by the International Economic Association at Tokyo,* edited by Mark Perlmann, pp. 162–73. New York: Wiley, 1974.

Fanara, Philip, Jr., and Warren Greenberg. "The Impact of Competition and Regulation on Blue Cross Enrollment of Nongroup Individuals." *Journal of Risk and Insurance* 52, no. 2 (June 1985): 185–98.

Farley, Dean E. "Competition among Hospitals: Market Structure and Its Relation to Utilization, Costs and Financial Position." Research note 7, Hospital Studies Program, U.S. Department of Health and Human Services, National Center for Health Services Research and Health Care Technology Assessment. 1985.

Farley, Dean E., and Christopher Hogan. "Case-Mix Specialization in the Market for Hospital Services." *Health Services Research* 25, no. 5 (December 1990): 757–83.

Farley, Pamela J., and Alan C. Monheit. "Selectivity in the Demand for Health Insurance and Health Care." *Advances in Health Economics and Health Services Research* 7 (1985): 231–48.

Feder, Judith. "Double Whammy for the Elderly." *Washington Post,* December 28, 1995.

Feldman, Roger, and James W. Begun. "The Effects of Advertising—Lessons from Optometry." *Journal of Human Resources* 13 supp. (1978): 247–62.

————. "The Welfare Cost of Quality Changes due to Professional Regulation." *Journal of Industrial Economics* 43, no. 1 (September 1985): 17–32.

Feldman, Roger, and Bryan Dowd. "Is There a Competitive Market for Hospital Services?" *Journal of Health Economics* 5, no. 3 (October 1986): 277–92.

————. "A New Estimate of the Welfare Loss of Excess Health Insurance." *American Economic Review* 81, no. 1 (March 1991): 297–301.

Feldman, Roger, and Warren Greenberg. "The Relation between the Blue Cross Share and the Blue Cross 'Discount' on Hospital Charges." *Journal of Risk and Insurance* 48 (1981): 235–46.

Feldman, Roger, Bryan Dowd, Michael Finch, and Steven Cassou. *Employer-based Health Insurance.* NCHR Research Report Series, DHHS Publication (PHS) 89-3434. Washington, D.C.: U.S. Department of Health and Human Services, June 1989.

Feldman, Roger, and Frank A. Sloan. "Competition among Physicians, Revisited." *Journal of Health Politics, Policy and Law,* Special issue on competition in the health care sector: ten years later, 13, no. 2 (summer 1988): 239–62. Reprinted in *Competition in the Health Care Sector: Ten Years Later,* edited by Warren Greenberg, pp. 17–40. Durham, N.C.: Duke University Press, 1988.

Feldman, Roger, Bryan Dowd, Don McCann, and Allan Johnson. "The Competitive Impact of Health Maintenance Organizations on Hospital Finances: An Exploratory Study." *Journal of Health Politics, Policy and Law* 10, no. 4 (winter 1986): 657–97.

Feldstein, Martin S. *Economic Analysis for Health Services Efficiency.* Amsterdam: North-Holland, 1968.

——. *The Rising Cost of Hospital Care.* Washington, D.C.: Information Resources Press, 1971a.

——. "Hospital Price Inflation: A Study of Nonprofit Price Dynamics." *American Economic Review* 61, no. 5 (December 1971b): 853–72.

——. "The Welfare Loss of Excess Health Insurance." *Journal of Political Economy* 81, no. 2 (March/April 1973): 251–80.

——. "Quality Change and the Demand for Hospital Care." *Econometrica* 45, no. 7 (October 1977): 1681–702.

Feldstein, Martin S., and Bernard S. Friedman. "Tax Subsidies, the Rational Demand for Insurance and the Health Care Crisis." *Journal of Public Economics* 7, no. 2 (April 1977): 155–78.

Feldstein, Martin S., and Kathleen Feldstein. "Stifling Health Care's Future." *Boston Globe,* September 21, 1993.

Feldstein, Paul J. *Health Associations and the Demand for Legislation: The Political Economy of Health.* Cambridge: Ballinger, 1977.

——. *Health Care Economics.* New York: Wiley, 1979.

——. "The Emergence of Market Competition in the U.S. Health Care System." *Health Policy* 6, no. 1 (1986): 1–2.

——. *The Politics of Health Legislation: An Economic Perspective.* Ann Arbor: Health Administration Press, 1988.

Finsinger, Jorg, Kornelius Kraft, and Mark V. Pauly. "Some Observations on Greater Competition in the German Health Insurance System for a U.S. Perspective." *Managerial and Decision Economics* 7 (1986): 155–61.

Folland, Sherman, Allen C. Goodman, and Miron Stano. *The Economics of Health and Health Care*. New York: Macmillan, 1993.

Foreman, Stephen Earl, John Anderson Wilson, and Richard M. Scheffler. "Monopoly, Monopsony and Contestability in Health Insurance: A Study of Blue Cross Plans." School of Public Health, University of California, Berkeley, October 1995.

Frank, Richard G., and David S. Salkever. "The Supply of Charity Services by Nonprofit Hospitals: Motives and Market Structure." *RAND Journal of Economics* 22, no. 3 (autumn 1991): 430–45.

Fraundorf, Kenneth C. "Organized Dentistry and the Pursuit of Entry Control." *Journal of Health Politics, Policy and Law* 8, no. 4 (winter 1984): 759–81.

Frech, H. E. III. "The Regulation of Health Insurance." Ph.D. diss., University of California, Los Angeles, 1974.

———. "Occupational Licensure and Health Care Productivity: The Issues and the Literature." In *Health Manpower and Productivity*, edited by John A. Rafferty, pp. 119–42. Lexington, Mass.: Heath, 1975.

———. "The Property Rights Theory of the Firm: Empirical Results from a Natural Experiment." *Journal of Political Economy* 84, no. 1 (February 1976): 142–43.

———. "Market Power in Health Insurance: Effects on Insurance and Medical Markets." *Journal of Industrial Economics* 27, no. 1 (September 1979): 55–72.

———. "Blue Cross, Blue Shield and Health Care Costs: A Review of the Economic Evidence." In *National Health Insurance: What Now, What Later, What Never*, edited by Mark V. Pauly, pp. 250–63. Washington, D.C.: American Enterprise Institute, 1980a.

———. "Health Insurance: Private, Mutual or Government." *Research in Law and Economics* supp. 1 (1980b): 61–73.

———. "The Market Power of York Hospital and the Damages Incurred by Dr. Weiss." Report submitted to the U.S. District Court for the Middle District of Pennsylvania, *Weiss v. York Hospital*, Civil No. 80-0134. August 8, 1985.

———. "Comments on (Hospital) Antitrust Issues." *Advances in Health Economics and Health Services Research* 7 (1987): 853–72.

———. "Monopoly in Health Insurance: The Economics of *Kartell v. Blue Shield of Massachusetts*." In *Health Care in America: The Political Economy of Hospitals and Health Insurance*, edited by H. E. Frech III, pp. 293–322. San Francisco: Pacific Research Institute for Public Policy, 1988a.

———. "Preferred Provider Organizations and Health Care Competition." In *Health Care in America: The Political Economy of Hospitals and Health Insurance*, edited by H. E. Frech III, pp. 353–72. San Francisco: Pacific Research Institute for Public Policy, 1988b.

———, editor. *Regulating Doctors' Fees: Competition, Benefits and Controls under Medicare.* Washington, D.C.: AEI Press, 1991.

Frech, H. E. III, and Paul B. Ginsburg. "Physician Pricing: Monopolistic or Competitive?" *Southern Economic Journal* 36, no. 2 (April 1972): 573–80.

———. "Optimal Scale in Medical Practice: A Survivor Analysis." *Journal of Business* 47, no. 1 (January 1974): 23–36.

———. "Imposed Health Insurance in Monopolistic Markets: A Theoretical Analysis." *Economic Inquiry* 13, no. 1 (March 1975): 55–70.

———. "Competition among Health Insurers." In *Competition in the Health Care Sector: Past, Present, and Future,* edited by Warren Greenberg, pp. 167–88. Proceedings of a conference sponsored by the Bureau of Economics, Federal Trade Commission, March 1978. Germantown, Md.: Aspen, 1978a.

———. *Public Health Insurance in Private Medical Markets: Some Problems of National Health Insurance.* Washington, D.C.: American Enterprise Institute, 1978b.

———. "Property Rights and Competition Health Insurance: Multiple Objectives for Nonprofit Firms." *Research in Law and Economics* 3 (1981): 155–72.

———. "Competition among Health Insurers, Revisited." *Journal of Health Politics, Policy and Law,* special issue on competition in the health care sector: ten years later, 13, no. 2 (summer 1988): 279–91. Reprinted in *Competition in the Health Care Sector: Ten Years Later,* edited by Warren Greenberg, pp. 57–79. Durham, N.C.: Duke University Press, 1988.

Frech, H. E. III, and Lee Rivers Mobley. "Resolving the Impasse on Hospital Scale Economies: A New Approach." *Applied Economics* 27 (1995): 286–96.

Frech, H. E. III, and J. Michael Woolley. "Consumer Information, Price and Nonprice Competition among Hospitals." In *Health Economics Worldwide: Conference Volume of the Second World Congress on Health Economics,* edited by Peter Zweifel and H. E. Frech III, pp. 217–44. Amsterdam: Kluwer, 1992.

Freeman, Howard E., Robert J. Blendon, Linda H. Aiken, Seymor Sudman, Connie F. Mullinix, and Christopher R. Corey. "Americans Report on Their Access to Health Care." *Health Affairs* 6, no. 1 (spring 1987): 6–19.

Freund, Deborah A., and Jay D. Shulman. "Regulation of the Professions: Results from Dentistry." *Advances in Health Economics and Health Services Research* 5 (1984): 161–80.

Friedman, Bernard, and Mark V. Pauly. "Cost Functions for a Service Firm with Variable Quality and Stochastic Demand: The Case of Hospitals." *Review of Economics and Statistics* 63, no. 4 (November 1981): 620–24.

Friedman, Milton. *Capitalism and Freedom*. Chicago: University of Chicago Press, 1962.

Friedman, Milton, and Simon Kuznets. *Income from Independent Professional Practice*. National Bureau of Economic Research no. 45. New York: NBER, 1954.

Fuchs, Victor R. *Who Shall Live: Health, Economics and Social Choice*. New York: Basic Books, 1974.

———. "The Supply of Surgeons and the Demand for Operations." *Journal of Human Resources* 13 supp. (1978): 35–56.

———. *The Health Economy*. Cambridge: Harvard University Press, 1986.

———. "The 'Competition Revolution' in Health Care." *Health Affairs* 7, no. 3 (summer 1988): 5–24.

Fuchs, Victor R., and Marcia Kramer. *Determinants of Expenditures for Physicians' Services in the United States 1948–1969*. New York: National Bureau of Economic Research, 1972.

Gelman, Judith R. *Competition and Health Planning: An Issues Paper*. Washington, D.C.: FTC, 1982.

Getzen, Thomas E. "A 'Brand Name Firm' Theory of Medical Group Practice." *Journal of Industrial Economics* 33, no. 2 (December 1984): 199–215.

Ginsburg, Paul B., Lauren B. LeRoy, and Glenn T. Hammons. "Medicare Physician Payment Reform." *Health Affairs* 9, no. 1 (spring 1990): 178–88.

Goldberg, Lawrence G., and Warren Greenberg. "The Effect of Physician-controlled Health Insurance: *U.S. v. Oregon State Medical Society*." *Journal of Health Politics, Policy and Law* 2, no. 1 (spring 1977a): 48–78.

———. *The Health Maintenance Organization and Its Effects on Competition*. Staff report, Federal Trade Commission, Bureau of Economics. Washington, D.C.: FTC, July 1977b.

———. "The Competitive Response of Blue Cross to the Health Maintenance Organization." *Economic Inquiry* 18, no. 1 (January 1980): 55–68.

———. "The Dominant Firm in Health Insurance: *Social Science and Medicine* 20, no. 7 (1985): 719–24.

Goldfarb v. Virginia State Bar, 421 U.S. 773 (1975).

Goodman, John C. "Health Insurance: States Can Help." *Wall Street Journal*, December 17, 1991.

———. "Second Opinion: Is the GOP Medicare Reform Just the Clinton Health Plan in Disguise?" *National Review* 47, no. 22 (November 27, 1995): 46–49.

Goodman, John C., and Gerald L. Musgrave. "Freedom of Choice in Health Insurance." National Center for Policy Analysis, Dallas, 1988.

Graddy, Elizabeth. "Interest Groups or the Public Interest—Why Do We Regulate Health Occupations?" *Journal of Health Politics, Policy and Law* 16, no. 1 (spring 1991a): 25–49.

———. "Toward a General Theory of Occupational Regulation." *Social Science Quarterly* 72 (December 1991b): 676–95.

Green, Larry. "Surgical Society's Rules Put Country Doctor in a Dilemma." *Los Angeles Times*, September 14, 1987, pt. 1, p. 20.

Greenspan, Nancy T., and Ronald J. Vogel. "An Econometric Analysis of the Effects of Regulation in the Private Health Insurance Market." *Journal of Risk and Insurance* 49, no. 1 (1982): 39–58.

Grosse, Robert N. "The Need for Health Planning." In *Regulating Health Facilities Construction*, edited by Clark C. Havighurst, pp. 27–32. Washington, D.C.: American Enterprise Institute, 1974.

Haas-Wilson, Deborah. "The Effect of Commercial Practice Restrictions: The Case of Optometry." *Journal of Law and Economics* 29, no. 1 (April 1986): 165–85.

———. "Consumer Information and Providers' Reputations: An Empirical Test in the Market for Psychotherapy." *Journal of Health Economics* 9, no. 3 (November 1990): 321–33.

Hadley, Jack, and Robert A. Berenson. "Seeking the Just Price: Construction of Relative Value Scales and Fee Schedules." *Annals of Internal Medicine* 106, no. 3 (March 1987): 461–66.

Hadley, Jack, and Robert Lee. "Toward a Physician Payment Policy: Evidence from the Economic Stabilization Program." *Policy Sciences* 10, no. 2 (December 1978): 105–20.

Hall, Thomas D., and Cotton M. Lindsay. "Medical Schools: Producers of What? Sellers to Whom?" *Journal of Law and Economics* 23, no. 1 (April 1980): 55–89.

Hamowy, Ronald. *Canadian Medicine: A Study in Restricted Entry.* Vancouver, British Columbia: Fraser Institute, 1984.

Harris, Jeffrey E. "Pricing Rules for Hospitals." *Bell Journal of Economics* 10, no. 1 (spring 1979): 224–43.

Havighurst, Clark C. "Professional Restraints on Innovation in Health Care Financing." *Duke Law Journal*, no. 2 (1978): 303–87.

———. "Doctors and Hospitals: An Antitrust Perspective on Traditional Relationships." *Duke Law Journal* 6 (1984): 1071–162.

———. "Explaining the Questionable Cost-Containment Record of Commercial Health Insurers." In *Health Care in America: The Political Economy of Hospitals and Health Insurance*, edited by H. E. Frech III, pp. 221–58. San Francisco: Pacific Research Institute for Public Policy, 1988.

———. "Are the Antitrust Agencies Overregulating Physician Networks?" School of Law, Duke University, November 13, 1995.

Havighurst, Clark C., and Philip C. Kissam. "The Antitrust Implications of Relative Value Studies in Medicine." *Journal of Health Politics, Policy and Law* 4, no. 1 (spring 1979): 48–86.

Hay, Joel W., and Michael J. Leahy. "Competition among Health Plans: Some Preliminary Evidence." *Southern Economic Journal* 50, no. 3 (January 1984): 831–46.

Headen, Alvin E., Jr. "Productivity Enhancing Customer Delay: Estimates from Physician Data Corrected for Measurement Error." *Southern Economic Journal* 58, no. 2 (Oct., 1991): 445–58.

Held, Phillip J., and Larry M. Manheim. "The Effect of Local Physician Supply on the Treatment of Hypertension in Quebec." In *The Target Income Hypothesis and Related Issues in Health Manpower Policy*, Bureau of Health Manpower, DHEW Publication (HRA) 80–27, pp. 44–59. Washington, D.C.: Department of Health, Education and Welfare, January 1980.

Hersch, Phillip L. "Competition, Regulation, and Hospital Behavior." Ph.D. diss., Ohio State University, 1982.

———. "Competition and the Performance of Hospital Markets." *Review of Industrial Organization* 1, no. 4 (winter 1984): 324–40.

Hixon, Jesse S., and Nina Mocniak. "The Aggregate Supplies and Demands of Physician and Dental Services." In *The Target Income Hypothesis and Related Issues in Health Manpower Policy*, Bureau of Health Manpower, DHEW Publication (HRA) 80–27, pp. 37–43. Washington, D.C.: Department of Health, Education and Welfare, January 1980.

Hoerger, Thomas J. " 'Profit' Variability in For-Profit and Not-for-Profit Hospitals." *Journal of Health Economics* 10, no. 3 (October 1991): 259–89.

Holahan, John. "Paying for Physician Services in State Medicaid Programs." *Health Care Financing Review* 5, no. 3 (spring 1984): 99–110.

Holt, Charles A., and David T. Scheffman. "Facilitating Practices: The Effects of Advance Notice and Best-Price Policies." *RAND Journal of Economics* 18, no. 2 (summer 1987): 187–97.

Hosek, Susan D., M. Susan Marquis, and Kenneth B. Wells. *Health Care Utilization in Employer Plans with Preferred Provider Organization Options*, R-3800-HHS/NIMH. Santa Monica: RAND, February 1991.

Hsiao, William C. "Public versus Private Administration of Health Insurance: A Study in Relative Economic Efficiency." *Economic Inquiry* 15, no. 4 (December 1978): 379–87.

Hsiao, William C., and Daniel Dunn. "The Resource-based Relative Value Scale for Pricing Physician's Services." In *Regulating Doctors' Fees: Competition, Controls, and Benefits under Medicare*, edited by H. E. Frech III, pp. 221–36. Washington, D.C.: AEI Press, 1991.

Hsiao, William C., and William B. Stason. "Toward Developing a Relative Value Scale for Medical and Surgical Services." *Health Care Fi-*

nancing Review 1, no. 2 (fall 1979): 23–38.

Huag, Marie. "The Sociological Approach to Self-Regulation." In *Regulation of the Professions: A Public-Policy Symposium*, edited by Roger D. Blair and Stephen Rubin, pp. 61–80. Lexington, Mass.: Lexington Books, 1980.

Huang, Lief-fu, and Richard N. Rosett. "Redistribution of Income through Blue Cross Community-Rated Premiums." Discussion Paper 72-9, Department of Economics, University of Rochester, June 1972.

Hughes, Edward F. X., Victor Fuchs, J. E. Jacoby, and E. W. Lewit. "Surgical Workloads in a Community Practice." *Surgery* 71, no. 3 (March 1972): 315–27.

Hyde, David R., and staff. "The American Medical Association: Power, Purpose and Politics in Organized Medicine." *Yale Law Journal* 63, no. 7 (May 1954): 938–1022.

Institute for Health Policy Solutions. *State Experiences with Community Rating and Related Reforms: Prepared for the Kaiser Family Foundation.* Waltham, Mass.: Heller School, Brandeis University, September 1995.

Jenkins, A. "Multiproduct Cost Analysis: Service and Case-Type Cost Equations for Ontario Hospitals." *Applied Economics* 12 (March 1980): 103–13.

Jensen, Gail A., and Jon R. Gabel. "State-mandated Benefits and the Small Firm's Decision to Offer Health Insurance." Working paper, Department of Economics, Wayne State University, July 1991.

Jensen, Gail A., and Michael A. Morrisey. "Group Health Insurance: A Hedonic Price Approach." *Review of Economics and Statistics* 72, no. 1 (February 1990): 38–44.

Johnson, Allan N., and David Aquilina. "The Impact of Health Maintenance Organizations and Competition on Hospitals in Minneapolis/St. Paul." *Journal of Health Politics, Policy and Law* 10, no. 4 (winter 1986): 659–74.

Joskow, Paul L. "The Effects of Competition and Regulation on Hospital Bed Supply and the Reservation Quality of the Hospital." *Bell Journal of Economics* 12, no. 2 (autumn 1982): 421–47.

Kartell v. Blue Shield of Massachusetts, U.S. Court of Appeals, First Circuit, 749 F. 2d 922 (1984a), p. 928.

Kartell v. Blue Shield of Massachusetts, U.S. District Court, District of Massachusetts, 582 F. Supp 734 (1984b), p. 755.

Kass, David I., and Paul A. Pautler. "Physician and Medical Society Influence on Blue Shield Plans: Effects on Physician Reimbursement." In *A New Approach to the Economics of Health Care*, edited by Mancur Olson, pp. 319–36. Washington, D.C.: American Enterprise Institute, 1981.

Keeler, Emmet B., Joseph P. Newhouse, and Charles E. Phelps. "Deductibles and the Demand for Medical Care Services." *Econometrica* 45, no. 3 (April 1973): 641–55.

Keeler, Theodore E. "Deregulation and Scale Economies in the U.S. Trucking Industry: An Econometric Extension to the Survivor Principle." *Journal of Law and Economics* 32, no. 2, pt. 1 (October 1989): 229–53.

Kendall, David. "GOP Resurrects 'Clinton Care.' " *Journal of Commerce,* November 1, 1995.

Kenkel, Donald. "Consumer Health Information and the Demand for Medical Care." *Review of Economics and Statistics* 72, no. 4 (November 1990): 587–95.

Kessel, Reuben. "Price Discrimination in Medicine." *Journal of Law and Economics* 1 (October 1958): 20–53.

Khandker, Rezaul K., and William G. Manning, "The Impact of Utilization Review on Costs and Utilization." In *Health Economics Worldwide: Conference Volume of the Second World Congress on Health Economics,* edited by Peter Zweifel and H. E. Frech III, pp. 47–62. Amsterdam: Kluwer, 1992.

Kinsley, Michael. "The Best Way to Fix Medicare." *Time,* September 4, 1995, pp. 24–29.

Klein, Benjamin, and Keith Leffler. "The Role of Market Forces in Assuring Contractual Performance." *Journal of Political Economy* 89, no. 4 (August 1981): 615–42.

Konold, Donald E. *A History of American Medical Ethics: 1847–1912.* Madison, Wisc.: State Historical Society of Wisconsin, 1962.

Kraft, Kornelius, and J. Matthias van der Schulenburg. "Co-insurance and Supplier-induced Demand in Medical Care." *Journal of Institutional and Theoretical Economics (Zeitschrift fur die gesamte Staatswissenschaft)* 142, no. 2 (June 1986): 360–79.

Kwoka, John E., Jr. "Advertising and the Price and Quality of Optometric Services." *American Economic Review* 74, no. 1 (March 1984): 211–16.

Lachs, Mark S., Jody L. Sindelar, and Ralph I. Horowitz. "The Forgiveness of Coinsurance: Charity or Cheating?" *New England Journal of Medicine* 322, no. 22 (May 31, 1990): 1599–602.

Landes, William M. *Affidavit: State of Maryland v. Blue Cross and Blue Shield Association.* United States District Court for the District of Maryland, Case HM 84-3839, May 15, 1986.

Lave, Judith R., Lester B. Lave, and L. Silberman. "Hospital Cost Estimation Controlling for Case-Mix." *Applied Economics* 4 (1972): 165–80.

Lave, Lester B. "An Empirical Approach to the Prisoners' Dilemma

Game." *Quarterly Journal of Economics* 76, no. 3 (August 1962): 424–36.

Lave, Lester B., and Judith R. Lave. "Hospital Cost Functions." *American Economic Review* 60, no. 3 (June 1970): 379–95.

Lee, Nancy Howell. *The Search for an Abortionist*. Chicago: University of Chicago Press, 1969.

Lee, Robert, and Jack Hadley. "The Supply of Physicians' Services to Public Medical Care Programs." Working Paper 1145-17. Washington, D.C.: Urban Institute, 1979.

Lee, Robert H., and Donald M. Waldman. "The Diffusion of Innovations in Hospitals." *Journal of Health Economics* 4, no. 4 (December 1985): 373–80.

Leffler, Keith B. "Physician Licensure: Competition and Monopoly in American Licensure." *Journal of Law and Economics* 21, no. 1 (April 1978): 165–88.

———. "*Arizona v. Maricopa County Medical Society:* Maximum Price Agreements in Markets with Insured Buyers." *Supreme Court Economic Review* 2 (1983): 187–211.

Leffler, Keith B., and Cotton M. Lindsay. "Markets for Medical Care and Medical Education: An Integrated Long-Run Approach." *Journal of Human Resources* 16, no. 1 (January 1981): 20–40.

Lefkowitz, Doris C., and Alan C. Monheit. *Health Insurance, Use of Health Services and Health Care Expenditures* (ACHPR Pub. 92-0017). National Medical Expenditures Survey Research F 12, Agency for Health Care Policy and Research. Rockville, Md.: Public Health Service, 1991.

Leland, Hayne E. "Quacks, Lemons and Licensing: A Theory of Minimum Quality Standards." *Journal of Political Economy* 87, no. 6 (December 1979): 1328–46.

Liang, J. Nellie, and Jonathan D. Ogur. *Restrictions on Dental Auxiliaries*, Bureau of Economics Staff Report. Washington, D.C.: Federal Trade Commission, May 1987.

Lindsey, Phoebe A. *State Laws and Regulations Governing Preferred Provider Organizations: Annotated Bibliography on Preferred Provider Organizations*. R-3442/3-HHS/FTC. Santa Monica: RAND, August 1986.

Lippincott, Ronald C. "Competition in the Health Sector: A Historical Perspective." *Journal of Health Politics, Policy and Law* 7, no. 2 (summer 1982): 460–87.

Lott, John. "An Open Letter to President Clinton from 565 Economists from all 50 States on Healthcare Reform." *Washington Post*, March 16, 1994.

Luce, R. Duncan, and Howard Raiffa. *Games and Decisions*. New York: Wiley, 1957.

Luft, Harold S., Deborah W. Garnick, David H. Mark, and Stephen J.

McPhee. *Hospital Volume, Physician Volume and Patient Outcomes: Assessing the Evidence.* Ann Arbor: Health Administration Press, 1990.

Luft, Harold S., Deborah W. Garnick, David H. Mark, Deborah Peltzman, Ciaran S. Phibbs, Erik Lichtenberg, and Stephen J. McPhee. "Does Quality Influence Choice of Hospital?" *Journal of the American Medical Association* 263, no. 21 (June 6, 1990): 2899–906.

Luft, Harold S., and Susan C. Maerki. "Competition Potential of Hospitals and Their Neighbors." *Contemporary Policy Issues* 3, no. 2 (winter 1984–1985): 89–102.

Luft, Harold S., Susan C. Maerki, James C. Robinson, Deborah W. Garnick, and Stephen J. McPhee. "The Role of Specialized Clinical Services in Competition among Hospitals." *Inquiry* 23, no. 1 (spring 1986): 83–94.

Luft, Harold S., Susan C. Maerki, and Joan B. Trauner. "The Competitive Effects of Health Maintenance Organizations: Another Look at the Evidence from Hawaii, Rochester, and Minneapolis/St. Paul." *Journal of Health Politics, Policy, and Law* 10, no. 4 (winter 1986): 625–58.

Lynk, William J. "Regulatory Control of the Membership of Corporate Boards of Directors: The Blue Shield Case." *Journal of Law and Economics* 24, no. 1 (April 1981): 159–73.

———. "Regulation and Competition: An Examination of the 'Consumer Choice Health Plan.' " *Journal of Health Politics, Policy and Law* 6, no. 4 (winter 1982): 625–36.

———. "Nonprofit Hospital Mergers and the Exercise of Market Power." *Journal of Law and Economics* 30, no. 2 (October 1995): 437–61.

Lynk, William J., and Michael A. Morrisey. "The Economic Basis of Hyde: Are Market Power and Exclusive Contracts Related?" *Journal of Law and Economics* 30, no. 2 (October 1987): 399–421.

MacIntyre, Duncan M. *Voluntary Health Insurance and Rate Making.* Ithaca: Cornell University Press, 1962.

Madrian, Brigitte C. "Employment-based Health Insurance and Job Mobility: Is There Evidence of Job-Lock." Working Paper 4476, National Bureau of Economic Research, September 1993.

Manning, Willard G. Personal communication. August 23, 1990.

Manning, Willard G., and M. Susan Marquis. *Health Insurance: The Trade-off between Risk Pooling and Moral Hazard.* R-3729-NCHSR. Santa Monica: RAND, December 1989.

Manning, Willard G., Joseph P. Newhouse, Naihua Duan, Emmit B. Keeler, Arleen Leibowitz, and M. Susan Marquis. "Health Insurance and the Demand for Medical Care: Evidence from a Randomized Experiment." *American Economic Review* 77, no. 3 (June 1987): 251–77.

Manser, Marilyn E., and Elisabeth A. Fineman. "The Impact of the NHSC on the Utilization of Physician Services and on Health Status in Rural Areas." *Journal of Human Resources* 18, no. 4 (fall 1983): 521–38.

Marder, William D., and Richard J. Wilke. "Comparisons of the Value of Physician Time by Specialty." In *Regulating Doctors' Fees: Competition, Controls, and Benefits under Medicare,* edited by H. E. Frech, III pp. 260–81. Washington, D.C.: AEI Press, 1991.

Marquis, M. Susan. "Cost-Sharing and Provider Choice." *Journal of Health Economics* 4, no. 2 (June 1985): 132–57.

Maurizi, Alex R. "The Impact of Regulation on Quality: The Case of California Contractors." In *Occupational Licensure and Regulation,* edited by Simon Rottenberg, pp. 26–35. Washington, D.C.: American Enterprise Institute, 1980.

Maurizi, Alex R., Ruth L. Moore, and Lawrence Shepard. "Competing for Professional Control: Professional Mix in the Eyeglasses Industry." *Journal of Law and Economics* 24, no. 2 (October 1981): 351–64.

Mayo, John W., and Deborah A. McFarland. "Regulation, Market Structure and Hospital Costs." *Southern Economic Journal* 56, no. 3 (January 1989): 559–69.

———. "Regulation, Market Structure and Hospital Costs: Reply." *Southern Economic Journal* 58, no. 2 (October 1991): 535–38.

McCarthy, Thomas R. "The Competitive Nature of the Primary-Care Physician Services Market." *Journal of Health Economics* 4, no. 2 (June 1985): 93–117.

McCombs, Jeffrey S. "Physician Treatment Decisions in a Multiple Treatment Model." *Journal of Health Economics* 3, no. 3 (December 1984): 144–71.

McGuire, Thomas G. "Patient's Trust and the Quality of Physicians." *Economic Inquiry* 21, no. 2 (April 1983): 203–22.

McLean, Robert A. "The Structure of the Market for Physicians' Services." *Health Services Research* 15 (fall 1980): 271–80.

Medical Staff of Doctors' Hospital of Prince Georges County. Consent Decree and Complaint, File No. 861-0143. November 30, 1988.

Melnick, Glenn A., and Jack Zwanziger. "Hospital Behavior under Competition and Cost-Containment Policies." *Journal of the American Medical Association* 260, no. 18 (November 11, 1989): 2669–75.

Mennemeyer, Stephen T. "Effects of Competition on Medicare Administrative Costs." *Journal of Health Economics* 3 (1984): 147–54.

Michigan State Medical Society. 101 F.T.C. 191 (1983).

Miles, John J. "Hospital Mergers and the Antitrust Laws: An Overview." *Antitrust Bulletin* 39, no. 2 (summer 1984): 253–99.

Misek, Glen I., and Roger A. Reynolds. "Effects of Regulation on the Hospital Industry." *Quarterly Review of Economics and Business* 22, no. 3 (autumn 1982): 66–80.

Mobley, Lee Rivers, and H. E. Frech III. "Firm Growth and Failure in Increasingly Competitive Markets: Theory and Application to Hospital Markets." *International Journal of the Economics of Business* 1, no. 1 (winter 1994): 77–93.

Monheit, Alan C., Michael M. Hagan, Marc L. Berk, and Pamela J. Farley. "The Employed Uninsured and the Role of Public Policy." *Inquiry* 22 (winter 1985): 348–64.

Moore, Thomas Gale. "The Purposes of Licensing." *Journal of Law and Economics* 4 (October 1961): 93–117.

Morrisey, Michael A., Frank A. Sloan, and Joseph Valvona. "Defining Geographic Markets for Hospital Care." *Law and Contemporary Problems* 51, no. 2 (spring 1988): 165–94.

Mulherin, J. Harold. "Complexity in Long-Term Contracts: An Analysis of Natural Gas Contractual Provisions." *Journal of Law, Economics and Organization* 2, no. 1 (spring 1986): 105–17.

Mullen, Patrick. "Kaiser, Other HMOs Adjusting Rates to Stay Competitive." *Medical Benefits* 6, no. 10 (May 30, 1989): 10.

Mullner, Ross, and Jack Hadley. "Interstate Variation in the Growth of Chain-owned Proprietary Hospitals: 1973–1982." *Inquiry* 21, no. 2 (summer 1984): 144–51.

National Association of Blue Shield Plans. *Membership Standards of the National Association of Blue Shield Plans.* Chicago: NABSP, May 1976.

Neipp, Joachim, and Richard Zeckhauser. "Persistence in the Choice of Health Plans." *Advances in Health Economics and Health Services Research* 6 (1985): 47–74.

Nelson, Charles R., and Richard Startz. "The Distribution of the Instrumental Variables Estimator and Its t-Ratio When the Instrument Is a Poor One." *Journal of Business* 63, no. 1, pt. 2 (January 1990): s125–s140.

Nelson, Phillip. "Information and Consumer Behavior." *Journal of Political Economy* 78, no. 2 (March/April 1970): 311–29.

Newhouse, Joseph P. "The Structure of Health Insurance and the Erosion of Competition in the Medical Marketplace." In *Competition in the Health Care Sector: Past, Present, and Future,* proceedings of a conference sponsored by the Bureau of Economics, Federal Trade Commission, March 1978, edited by Warren Greenberg, pp. 215–30. Germantown, Md.: Aspen, 1978.

———. "Commentary: Experience Abroad: Is It So Different?" In *A New Approach to the Economics of Health Care,* edited by Mancur Olson, pp. 202–10. Washington, D.C.: American Enterprise Institute, 1981.

———. "Is Competition the Answer?" *Journal of Health Economics* 1, no. 1 (June 1982): 109–16.

———. "Has the Erosion of the Medical Marketplace Ended?" *Journal of Health Politics, Policy and Law*, special issue on competition in the health care sector: ten years later, 13, no. 2 (summer 1988): 263–78. Reprinted in *Competition in the Health Care Sector: Ten Years Later*, edited by Warren Greenberg, pp. 41–56. Durham, N.C.: Duke University Press, 1988.

Newhouse, Joseph P., and the Insurance Experiment Group. *Free For All? Lessons from the RAND Health Insurance Experiment*. Cambridge: Harvard University Press, 1993.

Newhouse, Joseph P., and Charles E. Phelps. "New Estimates of Price and Income Elasticities of Medical Care Services." In *The Role of Health Insurance in the Health Services Sector*, edited by Richard N. Rosett, pp. 261–313. New York: National Bureau of Economic Research, 1976.

Newhouse, Joseph P., and Charles E. Phelps. "Price and Income Elasticities for Medical Care Services." In *The Economics of Health and Medical Care: Proceedings of a Conference Held by the International Economics Association at Toyko*, edited by Mark Perlman, pp. 139–61. New York: Wiley, 1974.

Newhouse, Joseph P., Charles E. Phelps, and M. Susan Marquis. "On Having Your Cake and Eating It Too." *Journal of Econometrics* 13, no. 3 (August 1980): 365–90.

Newhouse, Joseph P., and Vincent Taylor. "The Subsidy Problem in Hospital Insurance: A Proposal." *Journal of Business* 43, no. 4 (October 1970): 452–56.

Newhouse, Joseph P., and Vincent Taylor. "How Shall We Pay for Hospital Care?" *The Public Interest* 23 (spring 1971): 78–92.

Newhouse, Joseph P., Albert P. Williams, Bruce W. Bennett, and William B. Schwartz. "Does the Geographical Distribution of Physicians Reflect Market Failure?" *Bell Journal of Economics* 13, no. 2 (autumn 1982): 493–505.

Newhouse, Joseph P., Willard G. Manning, Carl N. Morris, Larry L. Or, Naihua Duan, Emmett B. Keeler, Arleen Leibowitz, Kent H. Marquis, M. Susan Marquis, Charles E. Phelps, and Robert H. Brook. "Some Interim Results from a Controlled Experiment in Health Insurance." *New England Journal of Medicine* 305, no. 25 (December 17, 1981): 1501–7.

Noether, Monica. "The Effect of Government Policy Changes on the Supply of Physicians: Expansion of a Competitive Fringe." *Journal of Law and Economics* 29, no. 2 (October 1986): 231–62.

———. *Competition among Hospitals*. Staff report, Bureau of Economics, Federal Trade Commission. Washington, D.C.: FTC, 1987.

———. "Competition among Hospitals." *Journal of Health Economics* 7, no. 3 (November 1988): 256–79.

Ocean State Physicians Health Plan, Inc., et al., v. Blue Cross & Blue Shield of Rhode Island, Federal Supplement 692, July 27, 1988: 52–75.

Olson, Mancur. "Introduction: A New Approach to the Economics of Health Care." In *A New Approach to the Economics of Health Care,* edited by Mancur Olson, pp. 1–28. Washington, D.C.: American Enterprise Institute, 1981a.

———, ed. *A New Approach to the Economics of Health Care.* Washington, D.C.: American Enterprise Institute, 1981b.

———. "Commentary: Organization and Financing of Medical Care." *Medical Care* 23, no. 5 (May 1985): 432–37.

Paul, Chris W. II. "Competition in the Medical Profession: An Application of the Economic Theory of Regulation." *Southern Economic Journal* 48, no. 3 (January 1982): 559–69.

Pauly, Mark V. "The Economics of Moral Hazard: Comment." *American Economic Review* 58, no. 3 (June 1968): 531–37.

———. "The Welfare Economics of Community Rating." *Journal of Risk and Insurance* 37, no. 3 (September 1970): 407–18.

———. *Medical Care at Public Expense.* New York: Praeger, 1971a.

———. "Indemnity Insurance for Health Care Efficiency." *Economic and Business Bulletin* 4, no. 4 (fall 1971b): 53–59.

———. "Overinsurance and Public Provision of Insurance: The Roles of Moral Hazard and Adverse Selection." *Quarterly Journal of Economics* 88, no. 1 (February 1974a): 44–62.

———. "The Behavior of Nonprofit Hospital Monopolies: Alternative Models of the Hospital." In *Regulating Health Facilities Construction,* edited by Clark C. Havighurst, pp. 143–62. Washington, D.C.: American Enterprise Institute, 1974b.

———. "Medical Staff Characteristics and Hospital Costs." *Journal of Human Resources* 13 supp. (1978): 77–114.

———. "The Ethics and Economics of Kickbacks and Fee-Splitting." *Bell Journal of Economics* 10, no. 1 (spring 1979): 344–52.

———. "Overinsurance: The Conceptual Issues." In *National Health Insurance: What Now, What Later, What Never,* edited by Mark V. Pauly, pp. 201–19. Washington, D.C.: American Enterprise Institute, 1980a.

———. *Doctors and Their Workshops: Economic Models of Physician Behavior.* NBER monograph. Chicago: University of Chicago Press, 1980b.

———. "What Is Adverse about Adverse Selection?" *Advances in Health Economics and Health Services Research* 6 (1985): 281–86.

———. "Taxation, Health Insurance and Market Failure in the Medical Economy." *Journal of Economic Literature* 24, no. 2 (June 1986): 629–75.

———. "Monopsony Power in Health Insurance: Thinking Straight While Standing on Your Head." *Journal of Health Economics* 6 (March 1987a): 73–81.

———. "Nonprofit Firms in Medical Markets." *American Economic Re-*

view 77, no. 2 (May 1987b): 257–62.

———. "A Primer on Competition in Medical Markets." In *Health Care in America: The Political Economy of Hospitals and Health Insurance*, edited by H. E. Frech III, pp. 27–71. San Francisco: Pacific Research Institute for Public Policy, 1988a.

———. "Competition in Health Insurance Markets." *Law and Contemporary Problems* 51, no. 2 (spring 1988b): 237–71.

———. "Market Power, Monopsony and Health Insurance Markets." *Journal of Health Economics* 7, no. 2 (June 1988c): 111–28.

———. "Fee Schedules and Utilization." In *Regulating Doctors' Fees: Competition, Controls, and Benefits under Medicare*, edited by H. E. Frech III, pp. 288–305. Washington, D.C.: AEI Press, 1991.

Pauly, Mark V., Patricia Danzon, Paul Feldstein, and John Hoff. "A Plan for 'Responsible National Health Insurance.' " *Health Affairs* 10, no. 1 (spring 1991): 5–25.

Pauly, Mark V., and David F. Drake. "Effect of Third-Party Methods of Reimbursement on Hospital Performance." In *Empirical Studies in Health Economics*, edited by Herbert E. Klarman (with Helen H. Jaszi), pp. 315–19. Baltimore: Johns Hopkins University Press, 1970.

Pauly, Mark V., and Gerald S. Goldstein. "Group Health Insurance as a Local Public Good." In *The Role of Health Insurance in the Health Services Sector*, Universities-National Bureau Conference Series, no. 27, edited by Richard N. Rosett, pp. 73–109. New York: National Bureau of Economic Research, 1976.

Pauly, Mark V., and Michael Redisch. "The Not-for-Profit Hospital as a Physicians' Cooperative." *American Economic Review* 63, no. 3 (March 1973): 87–99.

Pauly, Mark V., and Mark A. Satterthwaite. "The Pricing of Primary Care Physicians' Services: A Test of the Role of Consumer Information." *Bell Journal of Economics* 12, no. 2 (autumn 1981): 488–506.

Pertschuk, Michael. "Needs and Licenses." In *Occupational Licensure and Regulation*, edited by Simon Rottenberg, pp. 343–47. Washington, D.C.: American Enterprise Institute, 1980.

Pfizenmayer, Rickard. "Antitrust Law and Collective Physician Negotiations with Third Parties: The Relative Value Guide Object Lesson." *Journal of Health Politics, Policy and Law* 7, no. 1 (spring 1982): 128–62.

Phelps, Charles E. "Effects of Insurance on Demand for Medical Care." In *Equity in Health Services: Empirical Analyses in Social Policy*, edited by Ronald Andersen, Joanna Kravits, and Odin W. Anderson, pp. 105–30. Cambridge: Ballinger, 1977.

———. "Induced Demand—Can We Ever Know Its Extent?" *Journal of Health Economics* 5, no. 4 (December 1986): 355–65.

———. *Health Economics.* New York: Harper Collins, 1992.

Phelps, Charles E., and Joseph P. Newhouse. "Coinsurance, the Price of Time, and the Demand for Medical Services." *Review of Economics and Statistics* 56, no. 2 (August 1974): 334–42.

Phelps, Charles E., and Itai Sened. "Market Equilibria with Not-for-Profit Firms." Working Paper 191, Economics Department, University of Rochester, June 1989.

Phibbs, Ciaran, and Richard T. Carson. "Influences of Specific Clinical Services on the Shape of Hospital Market Areas." University of California, San Francisco, August 14, 1989.

Physician Payment Review Commission. *Annual Report to Congress.* Washington, D.C., various years.

Pope, Gregory C. "Hospital Nonprice Competition and Medicare Reimbursement Policy." *Journal of Health Economics* 8, no. 2 (June 1989): 147–72.

"Preferred Provider Organizations and Dentistry." *Journal of the American Dental Association* 107 (July 1983): 76–77.

Price, James R., and James W. Mays. "Selection and the Competitive Standing of Health Plans in a Multiple-Choice, Multiple-Insurer Market." *Advances in Health Economics and Health Services Research* 6 (1985): 127–147.

Ramsey, James B. "An Analysis of Competing Hypotheses of the Demand for and Supply of Physician Services." In *The Target Income Hypothesis and Related Issues in Health Manpower Policy,* Bureau of Health Manpower, DHEW Publication (HRA) 80–27, pp. 3–20. Washington, D.C.: Department of Health, Education and Welfare, January 1980.

Rappaport, John. "Diffusion of Technological Innovation among Nonprofit Firms: A Case Study of Radioisotopes in U.S. Hospitals." *Journal of Economics and Business* 30, no. 2 (winter 1978): 108–18.

Raskin, Richard D. "Of Messenger Models and Qualified Managed Care Plans: Implications of the St. Joseph and Danbury Consent Orders for Provider Networks and Antitrust Counsel." Chicago: Sidley and Austin, n.d.

Rayack, Elton. *Professional Power and American Medicine: The Economics of the American Medical Association.* New York: World, 1967.

Raymond, Harvey, Health Insurance Association of America. Personal communication, February 10, 1992.

Reed, Louis S., and William Carr. *The Benefit Structure of Private Health Insurance 1968.* USDHEW, Social Security Administration, Office of Research and Statistics, Research Report 32. Washington, D.C.: U.S. Government Printing Office, 1970.

Reinhardt, Ewe E. "Comment: Competition among Physicians." In *Competition in the Health Care Sector: Past, Present, and Future,* proceedings of a conference sponsored by the Bureau of Economics, Federal Trade Commission, March 1978, edited by Warren Greenberg, pp. 121–48. Germantown, Md.: Aspen, 1978.

———. "The Theory of Physician-induced Demand: Reflections after a Decade." *Journal of Health Economics* 4, no. 2 (June 1985): 187–94.

Relman, Arnold S. "What Market Values Are Doing to Medicine." *Atlantic* 269, no. 3 (March 1992): 98–106.

Rice, Thomas H. "The Impact of Changing Medicare Reimbursement Rates on Physician-induced Demand." *Medical Care* 21, no. 8 (August 1983): 803–15.

Rice, Thomas H., and Nelda McCall. "Factors Influencing Physician Assignment Decisions under Medicare." *Inquiry* 20, no. 1 (spring 1983): 45–56.

Robinson, James C. "The Impact of Hospital Market Structure on Patient Volume, Average Length of Stay and the Cost of Care." *Journal of Health Economics* 4, no. 2 (June 1985): 333–56.

———. "Hospital Quality Competition and the Economics of Imperfect Competition." *Milbank Quarterly* 66, no. 5 (1988): 465–81.

———. "HMO Market Penetration and Hospital Cost Inflation in California." *Journal of the American Medical Association* 266, no. 19 (November 20, 1991): 2719–923.

Robinson, James C., Deborah W. Garnick, and Stephen J. McPhee. "Market and Regulatory Influences on the Availability of Coronary Angioplasty and Bypass Surgery in U.S. Hospitals." *New England Journal of Medicine* 317, no. 2 (July 9, 1987): 85–90.

Robinson, James C., and Harold S. Luft. "The Impact of Hospital Market Structure on Patient Volume, Average Length of Stay, and the Cost of Care." *Journal of Health Economics* 4, no. 4 (December 1985): 333–56.

———. "Competition, Regulation and Hospital Costs." *Journal of the American Medical Association* 260, no. 18 (November 11, 1988): 2676–681.

Robinson, James C., and Ciaran Phibbs. "An Evaluation of Medicaid Selective Contracting in California." *Journal of Health Economics* 8, no. 4 (February 1990): 437–55.

Rogers, David. "House Committee Splits over Controls on Private Costs in Health Care Plan." *Wall Street Journal,* March 11, 1994.

Rogers, David, and Hilary Stout. "Health Care Reform Faces Deadlock in Congress as Lawmakers Wrangle over Rival Proposals." *Wall Street Journal,* February 25, 1994.

Rogers, James F., and Robert A. Musacchio. "Physician Acceptance of Medicare Patients on Assignment." *Journal of Health Economics* 2, no. 1 (March 1983): 55–73.

Romeo, Anthony A., Judith L. Wagner, and Robert H. Lee. "Prospective Reimbursement and the Diffusion of New Technologies in Hospitals." *Journal of Health Economics* 3, no. 1 (April 1984): 1–24.

Rorem, C. Rufus. *Affidavit of C. Rufus Rorem, Ph.D., C.P.A.*, presented to the U.S. District Court for the District of Maryland regarding *State of Maryland v. Blue Cross and Blue Shield Association, et al.*, Civil Action HM 84-3839, May 14, 1985.

Rossiter, Louis F., and Gail R. Wilensky. "Identification of Physician-induced Demand." *Journal of Human Resources* 19, no. 2 (1984): 231–44.

Rothschild, Michael, and Joseph Stiglitz. "Equilibrium in Competitive Insurance Markets: An Essay on the Economics of Imperfect Information." *Quarterly Journal of Economics* 90, no. 4 (November 1976): 630–49.

Rule, Charles F. "Antitrust Enforcement and Hospital Mergers: Safeguarding Emerging Price Competition." National Health Lawyers Association's eleventh annual seminar on antitrust in the health care field, Washington, D.C., January 21, 1988.

Russell, Louise B. *Technology in Hospitals: Medical Advances and Their Diffusion.* Washington D.C.: Brookings Institution, 1979.

Ryon, Ruth. "Governor Lifts Hospital Restrictions: New State Law Expected to Promote Construction." *Los Angeles Times*, October 7, 1984.

Salkever, David S. "Competition among Hospitals." In *Competition in the Health Care Sector: Past, Present, and Future*, proceedings of a conference sponsored by the Bureau of Economics, Federal Trade Commission, March 1978, edited by Warren Greenberg, pp. 149–62. Germantown, Md.: Aspen, 1978.

Salop, Steven C. "Practices That (Credibly) Facilitate Oligopoly Coordination." In *New Developments in the Analysis of Market Structure*, edited by Joseph E. Stiglitz and G. Frank Matthewson, pp. 265–93. Cambridge: MIT Press, 1986.

Satterthwaite, Mark A. "Consumer Information, Equilibrium Industry Price and the Number of Sellers." *Bell Journal of Economics* 10, no. 2 (autumn 1979): 472–82.

———. "Competition and Equilibrium as a Driving Force in the Health Services Sector." In *Managing the Service Economy*, edited by Robert P. Inman, pp. 239–67. Cambridge: Cambridge University Press, 1985.

Satterthwaite, Mark A., and David Dranove. "The Implications for Resource-based Relative Value Scales for Physicians' Fees, Incomes, and Specialty Choices." In *Regulating Doctors' Fees: Competition, Controls, and Benefits under Medicare*, edited by H. E. Frech III, pp. 52–70. Washington, D.C.: American Enterprise Institute, 1991.

Scherer, F. M. *Industrial Market Structure and Economic Performance.* Boston: Houghton-Mifflin, 1980.

Scism, Leslie. "Small-Business Program in California Cuts Health Premiums by Average 6.3%." *Wall Street Journal*, March 24, 1994.

Schlesinger, Mark. "Paying the Price: Medical Care, Minorities, and the

Newly Competitive Health Care System." *Milbank Quarterly* 65 supp. 2 (1987): 270–96.

Schlesinger, Mark, Judy Bentkover, David Blumenthal, Robert Musac- chio, and Janet Willer. "The Privatization of Health Care and Physi- cians' Perceptions of Access to Hospital Services." *Milbank Quarterly* 65, no. 1 (1987): 25–58.

Shalit, Sol. "A Doctor-Hospital Cartel Theory." *Journal of Business* 50, no. 1 (January 1977): 1–20.

Short, Pamela Farley, and Amy K. Taylor. "Premiums, Benefits, and Employee Choice of Health Insurance." *Journal of Health Economics* 8, no. 3 (December 1989): 293–311.

Shortell, Stephen M., and Edward F. X. Hughes. "The Effects of Regula- tion, Competition and Ownership on Mortality Rates among Hospi- tal Inpatients." *New England Journal of Medicine* 318, no. 17 (April 28, 1988): 1100–7.

Shryock, Richard Harrison. *Medical Licensing in America: 1850–1965.* Baltimore: Johns Hopkins University Press, 1967.

Sindelar, Jody L. "Disincentive Effects of Taxing Health Insurers." In- stitute for Social and Policy Studies, Yale University, July 1986.

———. "The Declining Price of Health Insurance." In *Health Care in America: The Political Economy of Hospitals and Health Insurance,* edited by H. E. Frech III, pp. 254–92. San Francisco: Pacific Research Insti- tute for Public Policy, 1988.

Sloan, Frank A. "Regulation and the Rising Cost of Hospital Care." *Review of Economics and Statistics* 63, no. 3 (November 1981): 479–87.

———. "The Effects of Health Insurance on Physician's Fees." *Journal of Human Resources* 17, no. 4 (December 1982): 533–57.

———. "Property Rights in the Hospital Industry." In *Health Care in America: The Political Economy of Hospitals and Health Insurance,* edited by H. E. Frech III, pp. 103–41. San Francisco: Pacific Research Insti- tute for Public Policy, 1988.

Sloan, Frank A., and Roger Feldman. "Competition among Physi- cians." In *Competition in the Health Care Sector: Past, Present, and Fu- ture,* Proceedings of a conference sponsored by the Bureau of Economics, Federal Trade Commission, March 1978, edited by War- ren Greenberg, pp. 45–102. Germantown, Md.: Aspen, 1978.

Sloan, Frank A., and Bruce Steinwald. "The Effects of Regulation on Hospital Costs and Input Use." *Journal of Law and Economics* 23, no. 1 (April 1980): 81–110.

Sloan, Frank A., Joseph Valvona, James M. Perrin, and Killard W. Ada- mache. "Diffusion of Surgical Technology." *Journal of Health Econom- ics* 5, no. 1 (April 1986): 31–61.

Spodick, David. "Effectiveness of Treatment: Mandating Appropriate Scientific, Behaviorial, and Ethical Standards—A Cardiologist Dissents." In *Dissent in Medicine: Nine Doctors Speak Out*, pp. 111–32. Chicago: Contemporary Books, 1985.

Stano, Miron. "A Further Analysis of the Physician Inducement Controversy." *Journal of Health Economics* 6, no. 3 (October 1987): 229–38.

Starr, Paul. *The Social Transformation of American Medicine.* New York: Basic Books, 1982.

State of Maryland v. Blue Cross and Blue Shield Association, Settlement Agreement. U.S. District Court for the District of Maryland, Case HM-84-3839, April 2, 1987.

Staten, Michael, William Dunkelberg, and John Umbeck. "Market Share and the Illusion of Power: Can Blue Cross Force Hospitals to Discount?" *Journal of Health Economics* 6 (1987): 43–58.

Stevens, Rosemary, and Jean Vermeulen. "Foreign-trained Physicians and American Medicine." Yale University, June 1971.

Stigler, George J. "The Economies of Scale." *Journal of Law and Economics* 1 (October 1958): 54–71.

———. *The Organization of Industry.* Homewood, Ill.: Irwin, 1968.

———. "The Theory of Regulation." *Bell Journal of Economics* 2, no. 1 (spring 1971): 3–21.

Stiglitz, Joseph E. "Competition and the Number of Firms in a Market: Are Duopolies More Competitive than Atomistic Markets?" *Journal of Political Economy* 95, no. 5 (October 1987): 1041–61.

Stone, Andrew G., Judith A. Moreland, John A. Johnson, Jill M. Brown, David M. Narrow, Barbara K. Shapiro, and Selig S. Merber. *Medical Participation in Control of Blue Shield and Certain Other Open-Panel Medical Prepayment Plans,* staff report to the Federal Trade Commission and Proposed Trade Regulation Rule. Washington, D.C.: FTC, Bureau of Competition, April 1979.

Svorny, Shirley V. "Physician Licensure: A New Approach to Examining the Role of Professional Interests." *Economic Inquiry* 25, no. 3 (July 1987): 497–509.

Telser, Lester G. *Competition, Collusion and Game Theory.* Chicago: Aldine-Atherton, 1972.

Temin, Peter. *Taking Your Medicine: Drug Regulation in the United States.* Cambridge, Harvard University Press, 1980.

———. "An Economic History of American Hospitals." In *Health Care in America: The Political Economy of Hospitals and Health Insurance,* edited by H. E. Frech III, pp. 75–102. San Francisco: Pacific Research Institute for Public Policy, 1988.

Thompson, John Larkin. "(Report) Prepared for Presentation to the Advisory Council on Social Security," April 6, 1983.

Thorndike, Nancy (Greenspan). "The Effects of Regulation in the Private Health Insurance Market." Master's thesis, University of North Carolina, 1976.

Tirole, Jean. *The Theory of Industrial Organization*. Cambridge: MIT Press, 1988.

Tseng, Kuo-Cheng. "Administrative Costs of Medicare Contractors: Blue Cross Plans versus Commercial Intermediaries." *Economic Inquiry* 15, no. 4 (December 1978): 371–78.

U.S. Bureau of the Census, *Statistical Abstract of the United States*. Washington, D.C.: U.S. Government Printing Office, various years.

U.S. Congressional Budget Office. *Physician Reimbursement under Medicare: Options for Change*. Washington, D.C.: CBO, April 1986.

———. *Physician Payment Reform under Medicare*. Washington, D.C.: CBO, April 1990.

———. *Rising Health Care Costs: Causes, Implications and Strategies*. Congressional Budget Office Study. Washington, D.C.: Superintendent of Documents, April 1991.

———. *The Tax Treatment of Employment-based Health Insurance*. Washington, D.C.: Congressional Budget Office, March 1994.

U.S. Department of Justice. "Merger Guidelines." (1992).

U.S. Department of Justice and Federal Trade Commission. "Statements of Enforcement Policy and Analytical Principles Relating to Health Care and Antitrust." DOJ and FTC (September 27, 1995).

U.S. General Accounting Office. *Health Insurance: Comparing Blue Cross and Blue Shield Plans with Commercial Insurers*. Report to the chairman, Subcommittee on Health, Committee on Ways and Means, House of Representatives, U.S. General Accounting Office, Report GAO/HRD-86-110. Washington, D.C.: GAU, July 1986.

United States v. the American Society of Anesthesiologists, 473 Supp. 147 (Southern District of New York) (1979).

van de Ven, Wynand, and Renee C. J. A. van Vliet. "How Can We Prevent Cream Skimming in a Competitive Health Insurance Market? The Great Challenge for the '90s." In *Health Economics Worldwide: Conference Volume of the Second World Congress on Health Economics*, edited by Peter Zweifel and H. E. Frech III, pp. 27–46. Amsterdam: Kluwer, 1992.

Vitaliano, Donald E. "On the Estimation of Hospital Cost Functions." *Journal of Health Economics* 6, no. 2 (June 1987): 305–18.

Vogel, Ronald J. "The Effects of Taxation on the Differential Efficiency of Nonprofit Health Insurers." *Economic Inquiry* 15, no. 4 (June 1977): 605–9.

Vogel, Ronald J., and Roger D. Blair. *Health Insurance Administrative Costs*. U.S. Department of Health, Education and Welfare, Social Security Administration, Office of Research and Statistics, Staff Paper 21, Washington, D.C., 1975a.

———. *Health Insurance Administration: An Economic Analysis*. Lexington, Mass.: Heath, Lexington, 1975b.

von der Schulenberg, J.-Matthias Graf. "The Effects of Government on the Region (sic) Market Structure of Physician Services." *Proceedings of the Forty-third Congress of the International Institute of Public Finance,* pp. 291–304. Detroit: Wayne State University Press, 1989.

Weisbrod, Burton A., and Mark Schlesinger. "Public, Private, Non-profit Ownership and the Response to Asymmetric Information: The Case of Nursing Homes." Discussion Paper 209, Center for Health Economics and Law, University of Wisconsin–Madison, December 1983.

Weiss v. York Hospital, 745 F. 2nd 786 814 3rd Circuit, 1984.

Welch, W. P. "Medicare Capitation Payments to HMOs in Light of Regression toward the Mean in Health Care Costs." *Advances in Health Economics and Health Services Research* 7 (1985): 75–96.

Werden, Gregory J. "The Limited Relevance of Patient Migration Data." *Journal of Health Economics* 8, no. 4 (February 1989): 363–76.

Wilensky, Gail R., and Louis F. Rossiter. "The Magnitude and Determinants of Physician-initiated Visits in the United States." In *Health, Economics and Health Economics: Proceedings of the World Congress on Health Economics, Leiden, The Netherlands, September 1980,* edited by Jacques van der Gaag and Mark Perlman, pp. 215–43. Amsterdam: North-Holland, 1981.

Williamson, Oliver E. *Corporate Control and Business Behavior.* Englewood Cliffs, N.J.: Prentice-Hall, 1970.

Wilson, George W., and Joseph M. Jadlow, "Competition, Profit Incentives, and Technical Efficiency in the Provision of Nuclear Medicine Services." *Bell Journal of Economics* 13, no. 2 (autumn 1982): 472–82.

Winslow, Ron. "Effort to Curb Health Costs Is Hitting Snags." *Wall Street Journal,* August 8, 1991.

Wolinsky, Fredric D., and Steven R. Steiber. "Salient Issues in Choosing a New Doctor." *Social Science and Medicine* 16, no. 7 (1982): 759–67.

Woolley, J. Michael. "Consumer Information and Competition among Hospitals." Ph.D. diss., University of California, Santa Barbara, November 1987.

———. "The Competitive Effects of Horizontal Mergers in the Hospital Industry." *Journal of Health Economics* 8, no. 3 (September 1989): 271–91.

———. "The Competitive Effects of Horizontal Mergers in the Hospital Industry: An Even Closer Look." *Journal of Health Economics* 10, no. 3 (October 1991): 373–78.

Woolley, J. Michael, and H. E. Frech III. "How Hospitals Compete: A Review of the Literature." *Journal of Law and Public Policy* 2, no. 1 (1988–1989): 57–79.

Wyszewianski, Leon, John Wheeler, and Avedis Donabedian. "Market-oriented Cost-Containment and the Quality of Care." *Milbank Memo-*

rial Fund Quarterly 60, no. 4 (1982): 518–50.

Zaretsky, Henry W. *Preliminary Results of Analysis of Modesto City Hospital and the Economic Impact of Its Acquisition.* Sacramento: Henry W. Zaretsky and Associates, 1984.

Zeckhauser, Richard. "Medical Insurance: A Case Study of the Trade-Off between Risk Spreading and Appropriate Incentives." *Journal of Economic Theory* 2 (March 1970): 10–26.

Zuckerman, Stephen, and John Holahan. "Medicare Balance Billing: Its Role in Physician Payment." In *Regulating Doctors' Fees: Competition, Controls, and Benefits under Medicare,* edited by H. E. Frech III, pp. 143–69. Washington, D.C.: AEI Press, 1991.

Zwanziger, Jack, and Glenn A. Melnick. "The Effects of Hospital Competition and the Medicare PPS Program on Hospital Costs in California." *Journal of Health Economics* 7, no. 3 (December 1988): 302–20.

Zweifel, Peter. *Bonus Options in Health Insurance.* Dordrecht: Kluwer Academic Publishers, 1992.

Index

About the Author

H. E. FRECH III is a professor of economics at the University of California, Santa Barbara. He has been a visiting professor at the University of Chicago and at Harvard University. From 1970 to 1972, he was an economist with the U.S. Department of Health, Education, and Welfare.

His current research focuses on health economics. Mr. Frech has published more than ninety articles and books. He is the North American editor for the *International Journal of the Economics of Business*, the series editor for "Health Economics and Public Policy" for Kluwer Academic Publishers, and a member of the editorial board of *Economic Inquiry*. He is also the editor and a contributor to *Regulating Doctors' Fees* (AEI Press, 1991).

Mr. Frech received his doctorate in economics from the University of California, Los Angeles. He is an adjunct scholar of the American Enterprise Institute.

A NOTE ON THE BOOK

This book was edited by Ann Petty of the
publications staff of the American Enterprise Institute.
The index was prepared by Nancy H. Rosenberg.
The text was set in Palatino, a typeface designed by
the twentieth-century Swiss designer Hermann Zapf.
Coghill Composition Company, of Richmond, Virginia,
set the type, and BookCrafters,
of Fredericksburg, Virginia, printed and bound the book,
using permanent acid-free paper.

The AEI PRESS is the publisher for the American Enterprise Institute for
Public Policy Research, 1150 17th Street, N.W., Washington, D.C. 20036; *Christopher DeMuth,* publisher; *Dana Lane,* director; *Ann Petty,* editor; *Leigh Tripoli,*
editor; *Cheryl Weissman, editor; Lisa Roman,* editorial assistant (rights and permissions).

DATE DUE

GAYLORD   PRINTED IN U.S.A.